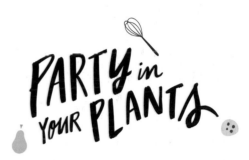

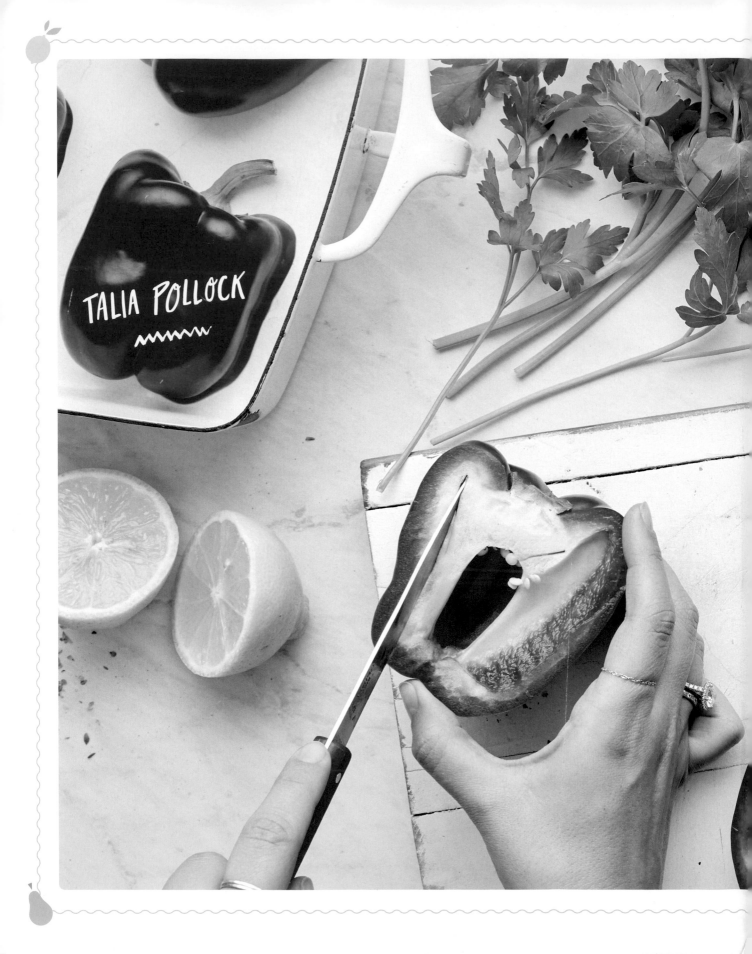

PARTY in YOUR PLANTS

100+
Plant-Based Recipes and Problem-Solving Strategies to Help You Eat Healthier

(Without Hating Your Life)

Avery • an imprint of Penguin Random House • New York

A
AVERY

an imprint of Penguin Random House LLC
penguinrandomhouse.com

Most Avery books are available at special quantity discounts for bulk purchase for sales promotions, premiums, fund-raising, and educational needs. Special books or book excerpts also can be created to fit specific needs. For details, write SpecialMarkets@penguinrandomhouse.com.

Library of Congress Cataloging-in-Publication Data
Names: Pollock, Talia, author.
Title: Party in your plants : 100+ plant-based recipes and problem-solving
    strategies to help you eat healthier (without hating your life) / Talia Pollock.
Description: New York : Avery, 2020. | Includes index.
Identifiers: LCCN 2019038469 (print) | LCCN 2019038470 (ebook) | ISBN 9780525540267 (trade paperback) |
    ISBN 9780525540274 (epub)
Subjects: LCSH: Vegan cooking. | Cooking (Natural foods) | Vegetarianism. | LCGFT: Cookbooks.
Classification: LCC TX837 .P6539 2020 (print) | LCC TX837 (ebook) | DDC 641.5/6362—dc23
LC record available at https://lccn.loc.gov/2019038469
LC ebook record available at https://lccn.loc.gov/2019038470
p.   cm.

Printed in China
10 9 8 7 6 5 4 3 2 1

Book design by Lorie Pagnozzi

TO ANYONE WHO'S EVER THOUGHT,
"HMM, I WONDER IF IT'S POSSIBLE TO FEEL A LITTLE
MORE AWESOME THAN I DO RIGHT NOW,
BUT I DON'T HAVE A PLAN. I DON'T EVEN HAVE A PLA—"
HERE'S YOUR PLAN. I WOULD OFFICIALLY LIKE TO EXTEND
TO YOU AN INVITATION TO THE PLANTS PARTY.

CONTENTS

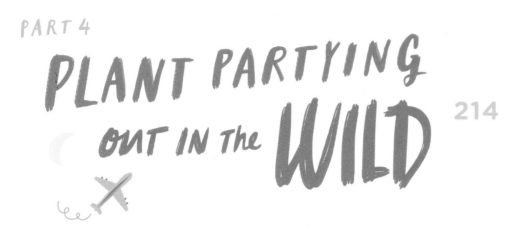

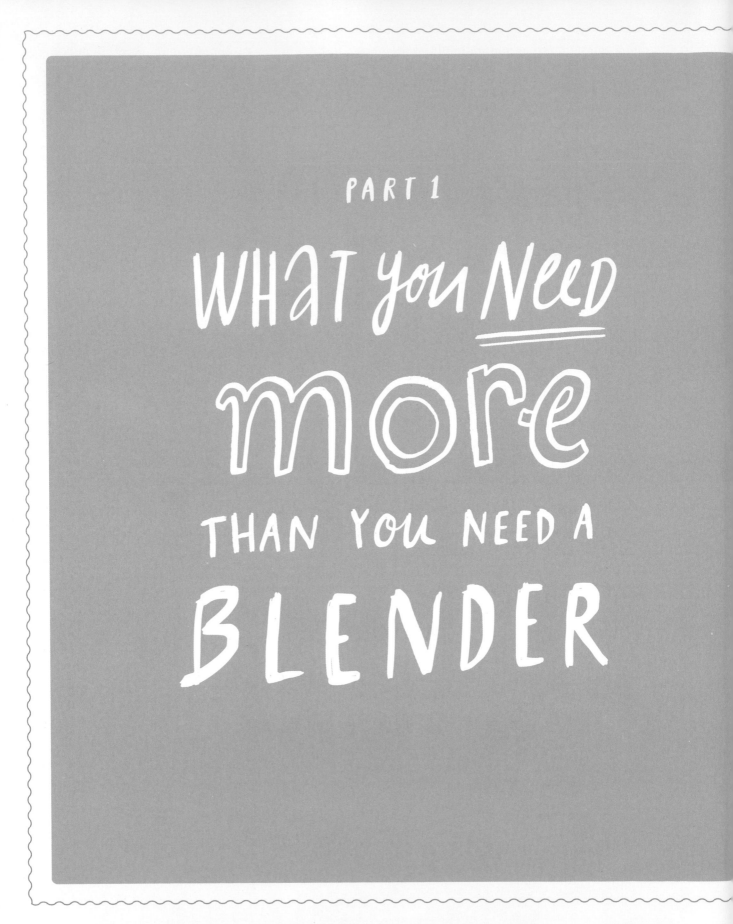

PART 1

WHAT you NEED more THAN YOU NEED A BLENDER

(but also why you need a blender)

You've bookmarked more healthy recipes than you could ever make in a lifetime.

Your shelves are overflowing with clean-eating cookbooks.

Your pantry has more superfoods than your closet has super clothes.

But you still can't get yourself to eat right on a regular basis. And you're constantly wondering, "What the h-e-double carrot sticks is wrong with me?"

I have good news. Nothing is wrong with you. You don't have a willpower deficiency. You won't benefit from another afternoon Pinteresting. And you don't need a fancy blender.[1] All you need is this book. And unless you're just "looking inside" online or turning physical pages in a real-life bookstore (in which case, cool! Take a selfie to show your grandkids), you already have this book, so your work is done.

---

1 Okay, you still kind of need a fancy blender. I mean, how else are you going to consume a bunch of plants in seconds so they taste good and make you feel and look good, too? This book, as life changing as I hope it will be for you, is not a 1:1 substitute for a blender the way that coconut sugar is a 1:1 substitute for regular sugar.

Seriously. Consider your "work" trying to eat healthfully done. Because, as you'll learn, healthy eating shouldn't and doesn't require "work." It doesn't require stress. In fact, stress kind of defeats the whole purpose. Healthy eating doesn't require suffering. Or a trust fund. It doesn't require a system. Or labeling yourself. Or a meal plan. Or tracking all your macros and micros and hippos. Or ashwagandha (unless you're into that).

But I know eating well is not always easy. Even though I'm a plant-based chef and wellness coach doesn't mean that heads of cauliflower neatly chop and wash themselves in my kitchen. Dinner doesn't appear on my plate. My dishes don't self-scrub. Healthy snacks don't pop into my pockets on plane rides. But I still manage to eat well *most of the time*. So I can feel and look my best most of the time. And so I can, ultimately, live my best possible life most of the time.

Because isn't that the point? Aren't we promised that, at the end of the apple-to-zucchini rainbow, there will be greater health, smaller pants, clearer skin, and endless positive energy? Well, that's all waiting for you. But tell me how you're going to enjoy all that good stuff if you're stressed out the wazoo, huh? If you're panicked over which phytonutrient to eat or worried about how Uncle Lou looked at you at the family barbecue as you picked up a veggie burger instead of his famous lamb chops. Who cares if you get sick less frequently or look amazing if you're white-knuckling through your kale salad?

I'll tell you this much: Your body sure as hell cares. Because stress is worse for you than french fries, FYI. That's why I'm going to teach you how to not eat Brussels with a bitch face. And that's why the only stress I support is stressing the importance of *not stressing* about healthy eating.

I'm really happy that you're here. Because what I've tried to do in my career is turn this whole it's-hard-to-eat-healthy umbrella inside out. And it's uncomfortable when umbrellas get turned inside out. You get wet, you cause a scene, you have to do that whole awkward backward hunch-over maneuver to turn it right side out. But, ultimately, an umbrella keeps you safe from the rain. And this book is going to keep you safe from a healthy diet ruining your life. Or a healthy diet being a thing you "sometimes do" when you're "being good" and "on track."

Enough with umbrellas. Let's party in your plants!

How to Read This Book

I've never understood why authors tell readers how to read their book. I mean, just continue to do what you're doing right now? Am I supposed to tell you, "If you read it upside down while wearing mismatching socks and listening to the *Friends* theme song backward and drinking a matcha latte, you'll crack a hidden code"?

Speaking of matcha lattes, did you know that, while one has about *three times* the amount of caffeine as a cup of green tea, matcha also contains L-theanine, an amino acid that chills your brain the heck out? So when the caffeine amps you up, the L-theanine swoops in there to take the edge off, and you're left energized but focused. Plus, matcha is super rich in antioxidants, which protect us from heart disease, high blood pressure, accelerated aging, inflammatory issues, and tissue damage. And it's high in an antioxidant called EGCG—kinda like BCBG, but instead of adorning our bodies, EGCG speeds up our metabolism and boosts our immunity.

If you're getting worried, like, "Talia, I don't want to over-caffeinate, plow through the first few chapters, and crash at Part Four," I'm here to tell you that in addition to the amazing stuff above, matcha also has antioxidants called "catechins," which *help stall the release of caffeine.* This means that the buzz comes at you gently, so instead of an energy spike you get a steady, all-day dose.

So how should you read this book? Maybe while sipping a matcha latte.

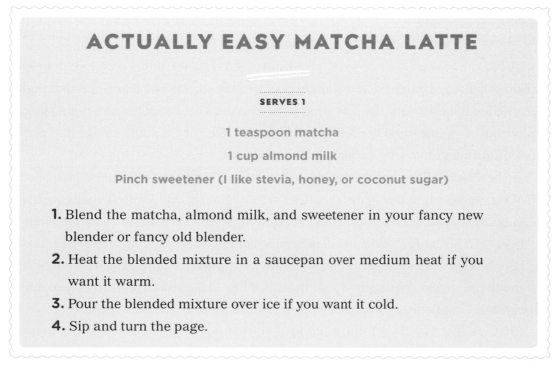

ACTUALLY EASY MATCHA LATTE

SERVES 1

1 teaspoon matcha

1 cup almond milk

Pinch sweetener (I like stevia, honey, or coconut sugar)

1. Blend the matcha, almond milk, and sweetener in your fancy new blender or fancy old blender.
2. Heat the blended mixture in a saucepan over medium heat if you want it warm.
3. Pour the blended mixture over ice if you want it cold.
4. Sip and turn the page.

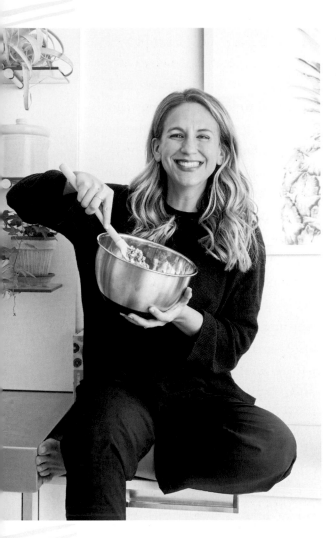

Who Am I to Tell You Anything?

#TBT TO THAT TIME PLANTS SAVED MY LIFE . . . THEN RUINED IT.

Five years ago, I was onstage in a sweaty NYC nightclub. I was also alone, with a microphone, trying to make people laugh as a stand-up comedian.

I told a funny story about my ex-boyfriend breaking up with me over a bacon burger (the same story you'll read on page 56, "True Life: I Got Cheeseburger Cheated On"). I joked about how annoying it is at concerts or festivals when omnivores get in the veggie burger line and clog up the works so us folks that *only* eat veggie burgers don't get the perk of a short line. I poked fun at people who told me, "I would literally die without cheese." (Statistically, there's only about a .3374 percent chance a lack of mozzarella sticks will end your life.)

I did stand-up a lot, and I always got a rush like no other when laughter and claps bookended my stories and jokes. But that night the reaction felt different. The following comedian did a set about her one-night stands and walks of shame—and the audience loved her. She got the same laughs and claps from the drunk crowd who had laughed and clapped for me.

All of a sudden it hit me. Hard. Like as hard as a $59 grocery bill from Whole Foods when you only bought five items. I realized in that moment that I wasn't changing lives with my silly-but-serious stories about healthy living—no more than that girl was changing lives with her stories about her debauchery. I didn't want to use my passion for making people laugh to get lip service from strangers. I wanted the things I said—even better if it made you giggle—to improve your quality of life. Make you happier. Give you more energy. More confidence. Fewer bellyaches. And fewer "stretchy pants" days.

That was the last time I did stand-up. I started my business, Party in My Plants, six months later with the mission of using humor to inspire people to eat more plants. And I wasn't trying to be some rando posting pictures of green food against a photogenic wall. I was already a certified holistic health coach, professionally trained chef, and expert in practical healthy living. In fact, I had changed my own life doing exactly what I now teach others to do.

Here's the thing: My life hasn't always been one big plant party. I stumbled upon this way of eating after years of feeling like total crap. For most of my life, I struggled with digestive distress, weight woes, immunity issues, chronic lack of energy, emotional problems, and a hell of a lot of anxiety. I sought out gastroenterologists, naturopathic doctors, acupuncturists, nutritionists, even a hypnotherapist. I tried every pill, test, supplement, herb, powder, and positive affirmation I could find. The best I got was an "IBS" diagnosis. (From my experience, a doctor telling you "it's IBS" really means "IDK," which makes "IBS" pretty much BS.) Eventually, I hit rock bottom. Which perhaps not coincidentally coincided with pooping in a bucket and snail-mailing that shit (literally) to a lab.

I figured I was fated for an entire life of bellyaches, binging, bloating, depression, and anxiety attacks. I saw myself feeling sick on my wedding day. Being too bloated to fit into my dress. Unable to eat my own cake. Forcing myself to dance because it was my wedding, dammit, but hunched over in pain in a bathtub "after party." I saw my hypothetical family of four trying to start a Sunday-morning-breakfast-in-bed tradition like my own family did growing up. I saw my hypothetical husband having to prepare specific food to accommodate my sensitive stomach and tell our kids to stop jumping on the bed not because the doctor said no more monkeys should do that, but because Mommy doesn't feel well. And I saw little Talia Jr. say sweetly but devastatingly under her breath, "Mommy *always* doesn't feel well." Too young to know that's bad grammar, but old enough to understand that her mother is a permanent buzzkill.

I really believed that was just the way it would always be.

That is, until one beautiful day in Santa Monica. I was a junior in college studying "abroad" in Los Angeles (coming from the East Coast, it really did feel like another country). I had gotten an internship at Adam Sandler's production company, Happy Madison, and my dream was to be a comedian. But all I was, was sick.

And so there I was in sunny California after a day on the set of *Rules of Engagement*, picking up my weekly bag of supplements from yet another place that promised to cure me. As I was checking out, I mentioned to the receptionist that I was hungry, and she suggested a place called Planet Raw for a coconut smoothie, which my belly would "love." When the dreadlocked dude brought me the creamy drink I had ordered,

I pushed it back and said, "I'm so sorry, but I don't do dairy." (I already wasn't "doing dairy" because I had proof in the form of alternating diarrhea and constipation that it pissed off my stomach.)

He said, "Oh no, sweetie, this smoothie is vegan."

I had no clue what vegan meant. This was in the dark ages before Beyoncé put it on the map. So, like a lactose-intolerant robot, I repeated, "I can't do dairy." But he insisted there was no dairy for me to do. I thought, "Everything I eat hurts my stomach anyway. What do I have to lose? YOLO!" (Except this was also before YOLO was a thing so I probably didn't think in that specific acronym.)

It was there, on that bench, amid a cloud of incense, that for the first time in over *eight years* I ate something that didn't make me feel awful. I didn't feel sick. No bellyache, no bloating, nothing.

I went back the next day. And the day after that. And the day after that day. When I wasn't eating this miracle food at this one woowoo establishment, I was sitting on the floor at Barnes & Noble transcribing recipes from vegan cookbooks onto a yellow legal pad. (This was before twelve-megapixel camera phones, pre–Prime shipping, pre–food blogs, and definitely pre-Talia having money to buy thirty cookbooks.[2])

I dove headfirst into the world of eating clean. I chugged the proverbial Kool-Aid—in this case, green juice. I cracked open coconuts with a machete. (This was *way* before coconut water was sold at gas stations.) I made my own almond milk. I went full throttle overnight, and it seemed like, overnight, all my health problems *disappeared*!

!!!!!

!!!

!!

But then so did my social life.

No way I could drink green juice *and* boxed wine, so I said sayonara to my sorority. I didn't eat gluten, meat, or dairy, but most restaurants weren't offering any alternatives, so I stopped eating out, which meant that I stopped going out with friends, and my family thought I was the most high-maintenance pain in the ass ever. The only thing I ever wanted to massage was kale, which meant my sex life went into the blender, too.

I had become a health nut hermit.

I was healthier than ever but unhappier than ever.

This was my second rock bottom.

But with every rock bottom comes a rock top. I set out to figure out how to balance

2 This feels like an opportune moment to interject with a big, fat, fully-loaded-with-coconut whipped cream THANK YOU for buying my book!

being both happy and healthy, so I no longer had to compromise one for the other. Because that's more BS right there.

Do we have to choose between a good hair day and a good work day?

Between good weather and good breath?

Between a good song and a good workout?

So why should we have to pick between feeling good and feeling happy? And, really, if we aren't both, we can eat all the damn spirulina we can find, but it won't matter because being miserable negates the benefits of the healthy stuff.

Oy. Talk about a catch-22 to the max.

So I went to the Natural Gourmet Institute to become a professionally trained plant-based chef, I obtained my holistic health coaching certification from the Institute of Integrative Nutrition, and I earned my certification in Plant-Based Nutrition through Cornell University. I was my first client.

And I was a great client. I learned to have fun at tailgates, road trips, ski vacations, beach vacations, casinos, music festivals, family dinners, and dates without neglecting my health.

Here's what I learned:

Are you ready?

This book. Everything I learned is in this book. That's why I wrote it! You've already heard that I went from sick to healthy, then healthy to unhappy, because the stress of giving up everything fun in life for the sake of sprouting my seeds started negating the effects of the living bacteria in my sprouted seeds.

If you take one thing away so far, it should be this:

you cannot eat brussels with a bitch face and expect to be healthy.

You must eat the Brussels with a smile (a real smile, not a family-photo-next-to-cousins-who-didn't-invite-you-to-their-beach-wedding smile) in order to reap the benefits.

In short, you must party in your plants.

All You Have to Do to Eat More Plants: A Brief Overview of This Book

I've been fortunate enough that hundreds of ladies—and some men! Hey, Kent!—from all over the world have actually traded their hard-earned (or well-gambled, I don't ask or judge) dollars for individualized help. I find that amazing, as a concept. I mean, I'm extremely grateful, but how are we living in a time where we need help doing something that we've been doing since we were dinosaurs or whatever? We need to eat in order to be alive, but very few of us know how to do that in a way that makes us *feel* alive.

For lack of a better and more intelligent term, it is whack that we don't know how to eat. But the struggle is real, and the solution is in your hands. I've reverse-engineered the process I've used to help all the people I've tutored over the years go from feeling truly unable to consume more healthy stuff to being as chill and routine with it as they are with their teeth brushing.

The first step in partying in your plants is to come clean about all the things about "clean eating" that suck cantaloupe balls. Things gotta suck before they get better, that's usually the way life goes. The only place to go is up. To a better place. Where you're eating well without extreme feats of willpower or extreme food FOMO.

The first step in partying in your plants is to come clean about all the things about "clean eating" that suck cantaloupe balls.

To get there, you have to come to terms with what parts of healthy eating are the peach pits—for you. Having kids who don't want to join you in your Pop-Tart embargo or a co-worker whose hobby is forcing people to eat her homemade eclairs aren't necessarily universal struggles. We have to name what exactly is coming between you and quinoa (or your personal culinary bugaboo) to get it out of the way. Also, let's be honest, there's nothing better than having someone validate your struggles. So that's what I'm here to do. Because your struggles are real and they can make healthy eating a bummer.

A warning: You might have to take responsibility for the times you've made life harder for yourself, too. Prepare to get honest and know that it's okay; I've done well-intentioned but ridiculous stuff, too. Like when I schlepped a Jack LaLanne juicer with me on a romantic vacation to a yurt in Big Sur with a boyfriend and spent way more time than I'm willing to admit washing, juicing, cleaning, and pooping than canoodling or relaxing.

The next step is to take the hell out of healthy eating at home. Unless you're a traveling salesperson or, I don't know, in the circus, you probably eat more often in your home than anywhere else, so it makes sense to focus there. We're going to get your kitchen, pantry, and fridge stocked like you mean business. Otherwise, you're not going to be able to make a healthy dinner at the end of a long-ass day, or prepare a healthy breakfast before a long-ass day, or pack a healthy snack for the middle of a long-ass day.

We'll talk about tools to make eating right a habit; we'll talk about meals that you can whip up in minutes, as well as recipes that are guaranteed to please picky family members. We're also going to visit the dusty devices in your kitchen that you definitely bought with the right intentions (or on the right Cyber Monday sale!) but definitely forgot about. Remember that spiralizer? Let's bring it back to life. Unlike old makeup, these gadgets don't expire, so let's get inspired, shall we?

A NOTE ON HOW RECIPES FIT INTO ALL THIS

Obviously, I can't advise you on how to eat without providing recipes. So this book has zillions of 'em. But they're not outlined by "morning, mains, spreads, snacks, and dessert." This is not just because I'm a rebel. It's because I believe that recipes out of context make less sense than recipes in context. Sure, a tasteful picture of basil avocado pasta is lovely, but seeing that basil avocado pasta in the context of "what to make when you're cooking for that cutie you swiped right for and you don't want to be too bloated to do *stuff* after dinner" brings it to life and helps you fit it into *your* life.

One of the things that my private clients get is the opportunity to ask for recommendations for their specific situations. But even though you and I aren't on the phone right now, I'm positive I've included recipes that you can use no matter what life throws your way. That's why the recipes here—all 100 percent plant based, gluten-free friendly (which means they'll smile at you *and* are easy to make gluten-free), and just-add-meat-able—are laid out within the bigger story about how to eat healthy stuff every day. Because you don't just need food for "morning, mains, spreads, snacks, and dessert," you need it for when you want to win the bake sale, cook for your Olive Garden–adoring husband, pack for a flight, fit into that Rent the Runway dress at your college roommate's wedding, and get over your hangover the next day.

Should You Get Jiggy Without Gluten?

I'm sure your mother taught you, "Don't just do what everyone else is doing. If everyone was jumping off the roof, does that mean that you'd jump off the roof, too?" But in the case of going gluten-free, it's worth considering following the crowd. It's not because ditching gluten is cool, and it's certainly not fun to annoy waiters at restaurants. It's because going gluten-free can be wonder-full.

The problem is, when people decide to go gluten-free, they often search for any replacement that's labeled "gluten-free." That's not the right way to start your gluten-less journey. A big reason this diet can be life changing is because when you cut out gluten, you cut out the majority of the processed food in your day-to-day. Switching to packaged gluten-free cookies and crackers may mean you're just eating *more* processed junk.

Okay, so what is gluten?

Gluten is a protein found in wheat, rye, and barley. It's what gives dough its elasticity and strength (it's derived from the Latin word for "glue").

The bagels that we get at the coffee shop are vastly different from the wheat our great-grandparents ate. That was the real deal—an unprocessed grain that gave them sustenance and a place to spread their homemade jam. It's a far cry to even call what we've got today wheat, which is why a lot of our bodies don't know what to do with it. Today's wheat is largely grown on mineral-depleted soil, from engineered seeds that are disease resistant but also less nutritious. After that wheat is harvested, it gets stored in silos for a long time, where it often gets contaminated with molds and fungi, and not in a kombucha kind of way. And when it gets baked into industrially produced bread, there's often extra gluten added to the dough to make it more elastic.

These days, wheat is one of the most common food allergies among Americans, in the top eight that make up 90 percent of all food-related allergic reactions. Its troublemaking protein can mean your liver has to work overtime to try to detox it. That toxic reaction (in which your body freaks out because it thinks you just ate poison) triggers your immune system to get all worked up, which can cause your intestinal tract to become inflamed, which can cause you pain.

It is quite possible (and even probable) that you have a gluten intolerance and don't know it. Some symptoms are obvious, like:

- abdominal pain after eating

- bloating and gas after eating

Other clues are less obvious, because they don't hit immediately. These sneaky signs can be:

- Foul-smelling poop (sorry to be blunt)

- Mouth sores

- Skin rashes

- Muscle cramps

- Joint pain

- Irritability

- Depression

- Diarrhea (randomly and regularly—not just after eating)

Generally, eating loads of glutenous grains (a.k.a. *processed* wheat) has a negative impact on your entire well-being. It can cause:

- crazy sugar and carb cravings

- weight gain and/or an inability to lose weight

- cellulite

- mood spikes

A recent study in the *New England Journal of Medicine* listed fifty-five diseases/ailments that can be caused by eating gluten. Things like:

- IBS (inflammatory bowel syndrome)

- inflammatory bowel disease

- cancer

- anemia

- osteoporosis

- regular fatigue

- canker sores

- rheumatoid arthritis

- MS (multiple sclerosis)

"But I don't have celiac disease. Should I still kiss gluten goodbye?!" you might be wondering. (Celiac disease is this type of inflammation and pain on a regular basis but on a much larger scale. If you have celiac disease you cannot—and should not—touch gluten with a twelve-foot pole.)

This is a listen-to-your-body situation (more on page 309). Cut it out for a week and see what's up in your body temple. If you feel even subtly more awesome than you did before giving gluten the cold shoulder, keep going for a month before reading your verdict to the judge.

Because I prioritize digestive ease over sluggishness, but because I don't have an intolerance or allergy, I eat a low-gluten diet. Do I panic if the only lunch place at the beach offers sandwiches? No. Do I cook and bake with gluten-free or low-gluten grains and flours? Yes. My faves, which you'll see in my recipes, are:

- brown rice (and brown rice flour)

- quinoa

- oats (these are often planted and/or processed alongside glutenous grains, so there's a risk of cross-contamination; if you're avoiding any traces of gluten, you'll have to buy labeled "gluten-free oats"; otherwise, you can just get the normal variety)

- almond flour (a.k.a. almond meal)

- chickpea flour

- spelt flour (which, note, does have gluten but is easier to digest for some folks with a mild intolerance)

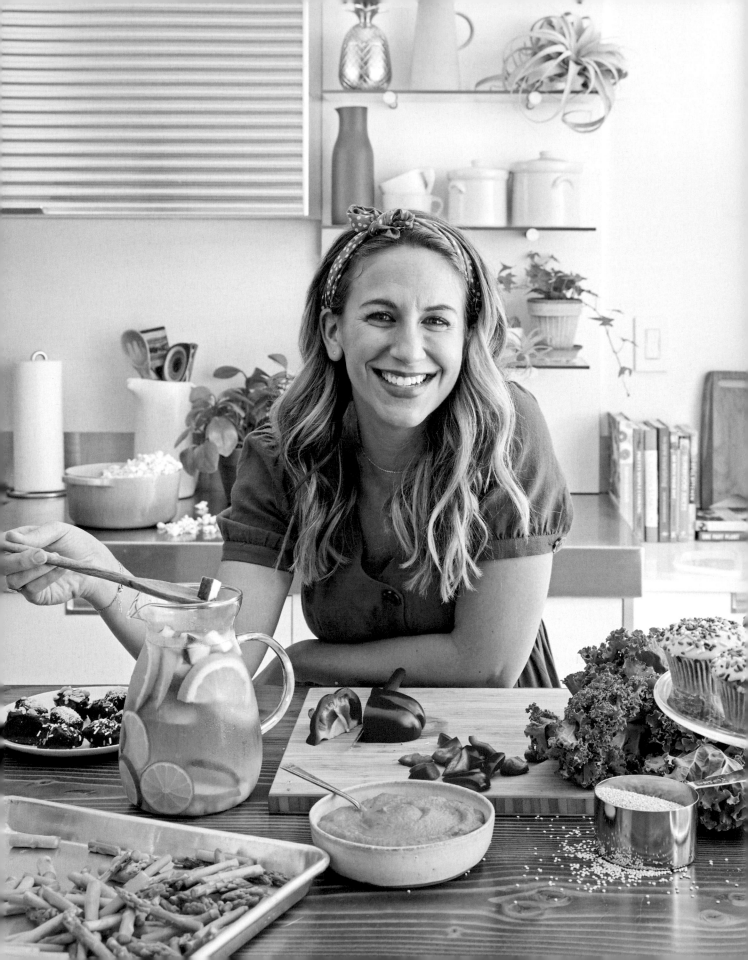

BACK TO: ALL YOU HAVE TO DO TO EAT MORE PLANTS

After we basically turn your home into Gwyneth's pantry, minus the ashwaganda, we're going to address the things that can still make healthy eating at home challenging. For starters, how about sharing your space with people who aren't into it at all? Which is why I'm going to teach you how to make "his and hers" meals (or "his and his" and "hers and hers" and whatever other gorgeous combination you embody).

It can be equally challenging to cook for yourself. If you live alone or are just flying solo for dinner, it can feel excessive or burdensome to make a full meal. Especially since one of my rules of thumb is that cooking time shouldn't be greater than eating time. We're going to talk about quick, simple meals that you can make while watching *Friends*, or how you can effortlessly turn frozen foods (not frozen pizzas) into warm, cozy feasts.

I'll also address the opposite of eating stag: entertaining. I love to throw parties, and your sexy new lifestyle doesn't mean forgoing hosting Thanksgiving or brunch—especially when you put my tips and recipes into action.

Finally, what else happens at home? Panic attacks over money. So we're also going to talk about eating on a budget and how to read labels and distinguish superfoods from super scams. You'll find recipes for making cheap veggies taste not so cheap and how to repurpose leftovers like a goddamn magician.

The next step is to get some fresh air. It's one thing to eat healthfully on your own turf (and that's hard enough), but it's a whole other thing to venture into the real world and master eating well in the land of fast food, expensive food, and food trends. Learn how to read between the lines of a laminated menu and communicate with your waiter in such a way that they don't want to spit in your food and you don't want to spit out your food. We'll cover traveling on planes, trains, automobiles, and feet; workplace eating; tailgating; picnicking; movie theatering; and more. By the end of this part you and healthy food will be like that Shakira song—wherever, whenever, you guys are meant to be together.

Finally, we'll tackle whatever is going on in your body. Healthy eating for its own sake is swell. But sometimes we want to be able to eat for specific purposes like losing weight, or fueling a workout, or improving your digestion, beating a cold, alleviating anxiety, and preventing big-picture diseases. Sometimes our body's purpose is to honor a chocolate craving—which I'm not going to tell you to fight but rather how to embrace it in a healthy way.

When you hit the chocolate recipes, you'll know you've made it. But to get to a place where your only struggle is choosing between cocoa and cacao, you first have to identify what's holding you back from eating apples instead of Apple Jacks.

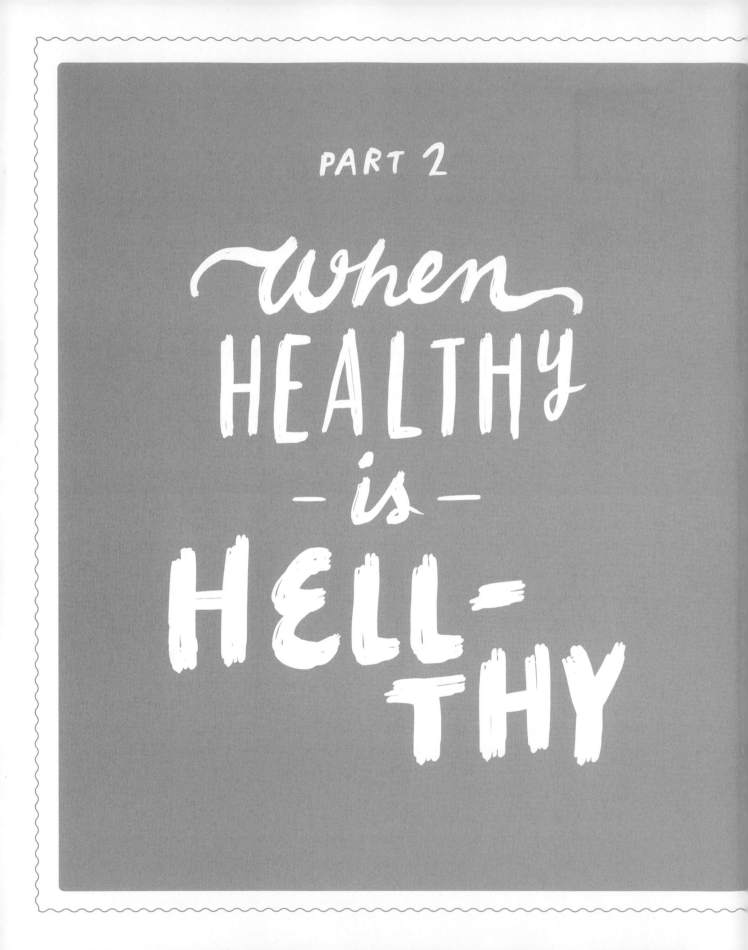

PART 2

When
HEALTHY
— is —
HELL-
THY

(and how to turn your clean-food frown upside down)

"Healthy eating" doesn't have a universal definition. Which sucks, by the way. How much easier would life be if "healthy" was like an outlet with one hole we could all plug into, and foreigners could simply buy a universal adapter. But it's more like headphone cords, which somehow *always* get tangled in seconds no matter *what we do*, causing chaos and stress and burden.

Luckily, in order to live a life wherein simply fixing a meal for yourself isn't as screwy as a headphone cord, I've created my own universal adapter:

Healthy eating = eating more plants* than you do crap.

(*in a given lifetime, year, week, day, meal, snack, drink . . .)

Everyone seems to swear by their specific diet, right? There are Zone fanatics and Whole 30 devotees, millions of people are reliant on Weight Watchers, committed to being paleo or vegan, vegetarian, pescatarian, lacto ovo, or octogono vegetarian. And while they may disagree on grains, oils, meat, dairy, and so on, they all have one thing in common.

PLANTS.

You will never meet a diet that doesn't encourage more plants. More produce. More veggies and fruits. Hell, Weight Watchers even *bribes* people to eat more plants—zero points, darling!

Focusing on eating more plants (and less crap) is the simplest and healthiest way to live. It's not about a label, not about rules, and has nothing to do with restriction. A plant-based diet also doesn't mean vegan, though it could. It doesn't mean paleo, though it could mean that, too.

It just means that the bulk of your diet comes from plants.

So what even are plants?

Plants are not made in a factory.

They are things that someone, maybe you but probably a farmer, planted.

They're the living colors that line the perimeter of the grocery store.

They grow mold, which is frustrating, but it just means they're alive. Which is a good thing.

They don't have pretty packaging, celebrity endorsements, or clever marketing slogans.

They're fruits, vegetables, nuts, seeds, legumes, whole grains, pure oils, and herbs.

And what is CRAP?

Crap is:

Chemical
Refined   **= CRAP**
Artificial
Processed

It comes in boxes, bags, or wrappers.

It flashes bright, well-branded labels like "natural!" "healthy!" "good source of fiber!" "whole grain!" "fresh!" "sugar-free!" "low fat!"

It's the snack that you find in the dusty box in your pantry and remember you bought it two years ago, but it hasn't aged at all.

It has ingredient lists longer than your grocery list, and includes words that sound made up, because those ingredients are made up . . . in a lab.

It's premade "food" you can open, heat, and eat now.

It's frozen dinners, bags of chips, boxes of cereals, baggies of baked goods, bars, bottles, cans, jars, and tubs.

Finally, what is plant-*based*? A plant-based diet means that the base of your diet is plants. Plants are what you mostly eat. It's the food group where most of your calories come from, the majority shareholder of the real estate on your plate, your shopping cart, your fridge, and your Instagram feed.

I can hear you wondering: Am I supposed to *only* eat plants?

I say: Only eat only plants if you want to.

Since plants are the most nutritionally dense stuff you can consume, the more absolutely the merrier, but that's not to say that there can't be room for cheese, cake (or cheesecake), chicken, or chips. Some call it "the 80/20 rule," but I don't like numbers—or rules—so I call it the "eat more plants than CRAP principle."

Your Body Can Handle Cheetos

One of the notions that trips people up is thinking that healthy eating means being "perfect." This is fake news! Healthy eating isn't an all-the-time thing; it's most of the time that matters most.

HEALTHY EATING 🍴
isn't an all-the-time thing;
it's most of the time
🍴 **that matters most.**

I tell the college students I speak to that they can still wind up with an A in a class even if they get some Bs and even a C.

I tell the clients I work with that it's still possible to win the Super Bowl if you lose some preseason games.

And I tell my mom that I am still an angel of a daughter even if I screamed "I HATE YOU!" more than once growing up, because true love is unconditional!

This all-or-nothing approach is a huge reason why healthy eating can feel like a raw deal. Thinking it's either nada or the full monty causes people to quit before they start, because who wants to make that choice about *anything*?

The truth is, our body can handle some Cheetos. Unless you have a specific allergy, your body can figure out what to do when it has to digest a little crap. Throughout this book (and for the rest of your life) I encourage you to simply focus on eating more plants than you do crap. Health and happiness will follow. It couldn't be simpler. But simple doesn't mean easy.

This is where my whole Party in Your Plants thing comes into play. I created Party in My Plants to make eating well as fun and as enjoyable and as non-sucky as a party. When you try it, you'll feel so fantastic that life will feel like a daily fiesta, too. Long gone are the days that eating healthfully had to be a drag. Those days haven't been the days since Ross and Rachel were on a break!

It's time to Party in Your Plants.

Much like I accidentally always leave my reusable shopping bags at home, I want to encourage you to intentionally leave your self-judgment and "why am I the worst?!"-ness out of all this.

For what it's worth: I'm not judging you, either.

When Healthy Is Hell-thy

If healthy eating was easy, obvious, inexpensive, and fun, you'd be doing it. I know that. You know that. Advertising agencies know that.

But healthy eating is often not easy, obvious, inexpensive, and fun. I also know that you also know that and advertising agencies *definitely* know that. Point being: I'm not sitting here on my high hempseed horse saying "WTF is wrong with you, it's so easy and dreamy to eat a pound of plants at every meal." I'm sitting here in my swivel chair with lumbar support telling you that you are 10,000 percent entitled to feel that it is a struggle. There's lots of pressure out there to feel that eating plants is NBD. I want you to know it *is* a big deal. Here's my empathy. Just take it. Put it in your pocket or your wallet or magnet it to your fridge.

Whenever I give a talk, I do a cliché-yet-effective thing: I say, "How many of you think, in some way, shape, or form, that healthy eating kind of sucks?" Every single person puts their arm up. I laugh and say, "Great. Well, I've made it my job to try to change your minds. That's going to be as easy as telling you that thigh gaps don't matter—or that Jell-O shots aren't fun." Which usually gets a roaring laugh when I'm speaking at a college (at that one women's church group, not so much—sorry, ladies).

The point is, it's not easy to convince anyone that Jell-O shots aren't fun so that's not my goal. I'm also not going to try to convince you that the things that make you feel like eating healthier is a burden/waste of your time/pain in the ass/embarrassing annoyance aren't real. I'm just going to say something my mama used to say to me, which is: "You can't complain if you can't explain." (At least, it *sounds* like something she would say when I'm grumbling about sorting my laundry by color.) So to my mama's hypothetical point: Let's explain that about which you complain.

"There's lots of pressure out there to feel that eating plants is NBD. I want you to know it is a big deal. Here's my empathy. Just take it. Put it in your pocket or your wallet or magnet it to your fridge."

GETTING CLEAR ABOUT WHAT PUTS THE "HELL" IN "HEALTHY EATING"

This section is intended to make you feel as good as that moment you come home from work and take off your bra. Or if you don't wear bras, it'll make you feel as good as that moment when you realize exactly what's been holding you back and are filled with so much clarity and peace and excitement that your best life is in plain sight. (If you didn't know, that's what it feels like to take off your bra.)

For the past five years, I've been collecting data. I ask everyone who comes across my website or who I meet in person or share an Uber pool with about their biggest hurdle when it comes to eating healthfully. From the thousands of brains I've picked,

I've come to some rad conclusions. First: When given the opportunity to vent about something we "should" be doing—and that we feel shame and frustration about not doing—it feels awesome. It can be amazing just to acknowledge your struggles and get them off your chest—much like a bra.

Here's the honest-to-god scientific truth: Eating healthy while you're unhappy about it benefits you about as much as expired sunscreen.

Second: It's not about the recipes. If you're like most of my clients, you probably already have a file full of photogenic meals that you'll never cook. The social stuff is much trickier—fitting new eating habits into already existent routines, work schedules, hobbies, passions, social circles, family culture. No one wants their life to revolve around their diet; rather, they want their diet to squeeze seamlessly into their full-to-the-max life. When healthy eating feels like a burden, you will not prioritize it over existent routines, hobbies, etc. And that's understandable. It's important. It's even essential. Because here's the honest-to-god scientific truth: Eating healthy while you're unhappy about it benefits you about as much as expired sunscreen. When healthy eating feels like hell, it causes inflammation in your body and disruption to your gut and diminishes your ability to digest and assimilate whatever you're eating—so it's ultimately a waste.

Unless you get clear on what's holding you back, you can bookmark all the pretty recipes you want and fill your produce drawers from the farmer's market—but you will continue to let those whoopie pies into your life.[3]

Is it hard when your co-workers bring in doughnuts? Does it stink when you're beat after a long day and your loved ones throw a fit when dinner includes color other than Kraft orange? Is it embarrassing to order on dates when you're self-conscious about seeming high-maintenance? Believe it or not, coming "clean" with yourself is the *only* step you need to take for smooth sailing into plant-packed paradise. I will catamaran you from there.

Know that it's normal for healthy eating to be a drag when you're first starting. Then turn the page for solutions.

---

3 What is the worst part about eating plants? Seriously. Go to www.partyinyourplants.com and tell me, right now, the number-one struggle you personally face when it comes to healthy eating. Don't hold back. Let 'er really, truthfully rip. Let your truth flow through your fingertips. (And I'll email you a copy for you to one day look back upon and reminisce about past woes.)

The Most Common "Hell-thy Eating" Struggles:

You are not an alien for feeling like healthy eating . . .

• Is so inconvenient that it feels wrong *not* stopping for fast food en route from work.

• Is not family-friendly when your kids will only eat veggies with a mountain of cheese or when your fiancé throws a fit if dinner doesn't include meat.

• Feels like mental and physical work, which, after a long day of work, simply does not work.

• Might result in couple's therapy because if forced to choose between you and chicken wings, bae would choose the wings.

• Takes the rest out of restaurants when you plead "Hold the butter" and just know the server is gonna roll his eyes.

• Ain't what you crave! You *want* to want plants like Jen Aniston wanted Vince Vaughn to *want* to do the dishes in *The Break-Up,* but you just gosh darn don't!

• Means meal planning, but you can't even remember to take your multivitamin, so how are you gonna prep a week's worth of lunches?

• Makes you feel like a sad sack at snack time. If you had more hours in the day, you'd make treats from scratch, but as it is your kids are inhaling processed snacks—and so are you.

• Doesn't sync up with your sweet tooth because fruit is not a dessert, thank you very much.

• Makes you feel like an ass for offending nice people like your boyfriend's sister, who wants to cook for you but is always making things you don't want to eat.

• Leads you to question your time management skills since every "easy" recipe takes longer than it should and the fact is if dinner prep is more than twenty minutes and uses a dozen bowls, it doesn't—and, really, cannot—happen.

• Has you questioning the meaning of life without cheese, so when your friends order that cheese plate or extra-cheese pizza, you partake—and suffer the consequences.

• Will put you on the streets since being thrifty seems nearly impossible. Why is crap food always the cheap food?

• Turns family events into a fiasco. While you'd feel more comfortable bringing your own dish, it's just so awkward with your future in-laws that you just eat the damn hot dog. And when you muster up the courage to bring vegan brownies for everyone, they treat it like a plate of celery.

• Can't coexist with alcohol. You love your friends and they love drinking. How are you supposed to honor your body temple without the boozy bonding?

• Makes Mom cry because she doesn't understand why you won't eat your childhood faves.

- Makes grocery shopping an inconvenient truth when you have to go to three different stores to get the ingredients you need.

- Means that, like the Girl Scout you never wanted to be, you always have to be prepared. Or else you'll fall back on the big Cs—carbs, cheese, and chocolate—which leads you to feel the other C: crappy.

- Paints you as "different." When you first went full veggie, your friends and fam were supportive, but then it became a "thing." They're trying to be sweet, but because everyone makes it a bigger deal than it is you end up feeling embarrassed. And even when your peeps accept your new habits, they make comments like "Hey, remember when you used to eat everything?"

- Is a snooze show. Like, after a while, all salads taste the same. You need the V in veggies to stand for variety!

- Constipates you. Period. Exclamation point!

- Is emotionally exhausting. It's easier to say "Yeah, let's grab wings after work" than "Actually, I packed a salad . . ."

- Becomes an unwanted obsession, which can be triggering for your prone-to-perfection self. The fear of failure, even with fruit, is real!

- Makes you feel deprived, which just makes you want it more.

- Equals TMI because the more you learn, the more stressed you get about what to eat. There's always some new study about what to eat or avoid. It's easier grabbing the sushi than spending the time figuring out if seaweed is a starch and if that makes it "bad."

- Makes you bitter because of those bitter greens. You just can't seem to make them taste good.

- Brings out all the judgy McJudgersons. It's hard to hear naysayers who believe that the very thing making you feel better is just "a fad."

- Feels impossible when it comes to staying consistent. You do so well for a while, but then you let loose and keep letting loose. Or you go through periods where you cook your heart out and others when you eat granola for lunch and dinner.

- Ain't a piece of cake when you can't bake a cake. You have no idea what to do with a sharp knife. Or your kitchen is generally stressful so you rush through making food and the whole thing feels unsatisfying—and then there's the cleanup.

- Makes you question your job because work gives out free breakfast, which is usually bagels, and even if you attempt to avoid the kitchen, you always get drawn in, and suddenly you've had two breakfasts and it's 10:00 a.m. Not only that, Kathy from marketing always has Snickers at her desk and that's hard to pass by.

HOW HEALTHY EATING IS LIKE A HAIRY SHOWER DRAIN: AN ANALOGY THAT'LL HOPEFULLY STICK WITH YOU

I once lived in a prewar five-floor walk-up in lower Manhattan. The floor number isn't relevant, but I want to paint a picture. To keep that picture painted, you should know that my apartment was the smallest apartment known to man: too small to fit a bed frame *and* a dresser, so my mattress was on the floor. I was able to wash dishes, go to sleep, brush my teeth, cook, eat, and watch TV all without picking up my pivot foot. Again, not really relevant, but stick with me.

My shower had one of those old drains without a cover or a stopper or anything; it was just an open hole. But after living in this 120-square-foot apartment for a few months, that hole wasn't so open. When I showered, the tub would fill with water. Even though my toe hairs (c'mon! We all have them!) were enjoying the extra conditioning from that soapy H_2O, I was completely grossed out about showering ankle-deep in muck. I knew I had to unclog the drain. But I also knew that I'd rather pull a full Britney Spears head shave than go into my pre-electricity-era drain and pull out globs of moldy hair from the 1800s (I'm currently gagging just thinking about it), so I just miserably showered knee-deep for the next eight months until it got fixed. And by "got fixed," I mean I moved.

This is all to say that if we hate doing things, even if the consequences of not doing those things mean we're showering in yucky water that makes you want to die, we still won't do those things. If you don't enjoy eating a certain way, damn straight you won't do it. I mean, you're talking to a person who almost flooded her apartment just to avoid what had to happen. So if you're not eating healthfully with ease and or with joy right now, or if just reading "healthy eating sucks" gives you a butterfly or two in your stomach because it's your honest-to-god truth, then accept it. It's only once you're able to come out of the clean-food-isn't-enjoyable closet that we can identify why that is, and hire a plumber—oops, I got my analogies mixed up. We can find solutions that'll actually work.

So let's get clear.

YOU CAN'T WHITE-KNUCKLE KALE

I've been harping on this whole "the benefits of healthy eating don't outweigh the stress of it," huh? That's partially because I want you to be a happy person who doesn't resent something that can radically level-up your life. And, yeah, because willpower studies have proven that if something sucks you will not stick with it, no matter how much gusto you start with. But the real reason is because when we eat while angry, resentful, anxious, or in any negative emotional state, we impair our body's ability to take in that wholesome stuff and do something worthwhile with it. If you white-knuckle kale, you're negating the benefits of that kale.

No joke, stress is worse for you than deep-fried cheese. Which is why I always tell people that I'd rather they eat deep-fried cheese sticks with a smile than Brussels sprouts with a bitch face.

Surely you've heard aphorisms like "Don't eat while standing up," "Don't eat while walking," or "Don't eat when you're upset." It's been said[4] that the gut is the seat of emotion, and the research confirms that it's basically a second brain. After the brain in your head, your gut has the largest bundle of nerves in your body—over 100 million neurons hustling inside your intestinal wall. And much like your brain sends signals to the rest of your body, your gut DMs your brain about how everything's going on the flip side of your belly button. When your brain is stressed or anxious, its midriff BFF shuts down its digestive capabilities to allow more blood flow to potentially flee or fight.

If you're feeling anxious about whether your kids will eat cauliflower tonight, resentful that your co-workers get to have Mindy's maternity-leave-party ice cream cake and you don't, cursing the world because you're spending your weekend meal prepping instead of playing golf—whatever it is, those negative emotions are worse for you than a doughnut. Even half a doughnut. Hell, they're probably worse for you than a doughnut hole. If your digestive system is on hiatus because it thinks you need that blood flow elsewhere (even though you're just thinking about how much you'd rather be eating a BLT than just a T), the food you're eating, 'scuze me, the *food you're eating resentfully*, can fly through your system way too quickly to give the nutrients a chance to be absorbed and let you reap the benefits. Which makes the whole "healthy eating thing" almost pointless.

I once read that stress is "an acute threat to homeostasis."[5] Homeostasis is inner peace, when your inner state is chilling in equilibrium and health. Stress knocks that well-being out of balance. And chronic stress has a significant effect on our immune system, too.

Rather than continuing to freak you out, I'm going to assume you get the point, right? Eating healthy while pissed is close to pointless.

---

4 By Johann Wolfgang von Goethe, the great German writer and philosopher, duh.

5 Chuong, RS and Talley, NJ. "Epidemiology and clinical presentation of stress-related peptic damage and chronic peptic ulcer," *Curr Mol Med*, June 2008, 8(4): 253–257.

Let's Also Admit That Eating Not Healthy Sucks, Too

So, eating healthy can be annoying, inconvenient, stressful, and a burden. But what about how *not* eating healthy can be a downer as well? After all, there are two sides to every story, and every coin—and every cucumber slice.

Maybe one of these sounds familiar:

• Lacking the energy to play kickball with your kids (or too sluggish to play Scrabble with your nerdy kids).

• Feeling foggy in your brain.

• Seeing everything, even full glasses, as half empty. Because you're depressed.

• Living every day in your "fat day" jeans.

• Picking up every cold, cough, and sniffle in a one-block radius because your immune system sucks.

• Needing to wear makeup to cover up all sorts of skin problems.

• Looking years older than you are.

• Dealing with weak, brittle hair and nails that mimic crackers. Because they crack a lot and aren't shiny.

• Flirting with heart disease, diabetes, and blood pressure and cholesterol as high as Chevy Chase's Christmas tree in *National Lampoon's Christmas Vacation*. You know—the one that busts through the living-room ceiling.

• Pooping about as frequently as you do laundry. (Nobody does laundry every day, right? Usually like once a week?)

• Feeling your blood sugar seesaw crazier than a kid on an actual seesaw.

• Not being able to remember the last time you slept through the night or woke up well-rested.

• Falling asleep at your desk, your dinner table, or your kid's dance recital. (To be fair, even the healthiest eater is likely to fall asleep at a kid's dance recital, but the dinner table or desk is a red flag.)

• Not playing your hobby sports (whether it's golf, tennis, skiing, snowboarding, jogging, or yoga-ing) as athletically as you know you can or want to. Your bones are weak and your joints need a dose of WD-40.

• Same as the above, just sub "sex" for golf.

• Feeling under the sway of your cravings.

• Relying on Tic Tacs, mouthwash, gum, or antisocial tendencies to mask your persistent stanky breath.

• Being a living, walking, hyperventilating billboard for anxiety.

Just because someone fits into sample sizes doesn't mean they're not experiencing the negative effects of eating crap in invisible-to-you ways.

We've got ourselves into a dill pickle here: Healthy eating can be a buzzkill, but not eating healthy can just kill you. Sorry if that sounds dramatic, but it's true: It can increase your risk for cancer, diabetes, heart disease, obesity, stroke, and Alzheimer's—in addition to just making your day-to-day life harder than it needs to be.

Somewhere along the way, we lumped together a healthy inside with a skinny outside like the dancing twin emoji girls. But wearing size-zero pants doesn't mean you eat enough plants. And eating plants doesn't mean you wear zero pants—I mean, size-zero pants.

I know this is a depressingly normal thought process because I've been there, and I've heard it from nearly every woman I've coached or casually spoken to in a grocery store line.

"Why am I stuck eating a salad, seasoning it with my tears, while my bestie chomps down pizza, burgers, and milk shakes and stays so thin?"

"My office is loaded with junk food and my co-workers stay skinny even though they down bags of chips; if I try that, I inflate like a balloon."

Look, just because someone fits into sample sizes doesn't mean they're not experiencing the negative effects of eating crap in invisible-to-you ways. You can't see high blood pressure. And if *you're* the one able to eat whatever the heck you want and still fit into your prom dress, it doesn't mean you don't also need to pay attention.

A top-notch diet can help you find a happy, comfortable weight, but it's not necessarily a weight-loss diet. Instead, it's the permanent route to feeling, looking, thinking, and living your best life.

YOU DON'T KNOW THE GLOW YOU DON'T KNOW

Nicole started working with me to, in her words, "lose weight, stop body shaming myself and get my independence with food choices back." She had so much anxiety, guilt, and stress associated with food that she felt terrible about everything she ate while believing that nothing she did was good enough. Even though she knew it caused a ruckus in her gut-kus, she ate ice cream and red meat and made frequent stops at Chipotle and Chick-fil-A. When she got stressed she'd have an extra glass of wine, get a lil lazy, and make indulgent choices that she later regretted.

She needed help getting back to a lifestyle that would allow her to "finally get her body and happiness back." We talked about ways to comfortably eat more plants and less crap, starting with a simple morning routine: waking up, making a smoothie, sweating, showering, and chilling with a plant protein–packed breakfast.

We craving-clenching welcomed banana ice cream (page 110), after a low-stress dinner (page 105). We swapped highly processed bread for a hearty sprouted bread—perfect for snacks of avocado toast or nut butter toast with blueberries or apple. I aimed to empower her to feel the joy of consistency.

Six days later, I got a text from Nicole saying that she had so much energy it was "unreal." She couldn't stop smiling and talking and was worried about coming across as obnoxiously chipper. She was glowing. Her co-workers asked if she was seeing someone new.

A couple of months later, Nicole was still going strong—not because I sent her some superhuman willpower via my smartphone but because she now knew how incredible she *could* feel. She had no idea that along the journey, she'd stumble upon a stockpile of energy that made her question how she had been able to live all her twenty-eight years prior without it.

Your Plan to Party in Your Plants

You can't have (or spell) a plant party without "plan."

It's like how you can't have a charged phone without a phone charger. The last thing you want is for your phone to die while you're out 'n' about living your life. So you take 3.9 seconds to grab your charger and stick it in your bag (plus bonus a battery in your pocket).

That's not a burden, right, to plan how you'll keep your battery charged? The same logic applies to eating better. The first thing to do—which will also help you keep track of how much better you feel after you learn to Party in Your Plants—is to write down the specific ways you think your crummy diet is affecting you.

Get out a piece of paper or your Notes app and list them out right now. Write what happens when you eat crappy foods, when you don't take care of yourself, when the only plant you eat all day is a tomato on your tuna salad sandwich. Then make a list of all of the amazing things that happen when you eat right.

I'll bet my Vitamix that if you can consistently remind yourself of the negative stuff that happens when you don't eat well and the positive stuff that happens when you incorporate more plants, you'll be able to make a lasting change as easily and automatically as keeping your phone charged. Just like you might buy a portable backup charger do-hickey, keep a spare charger in your purse, or place your phone on low battery mode to keep it running, this book is packed with plant-eating do-hickeys, spare plants you can keep in your purse, and clever tricks that'll help you eat great—and feel even better.

Let's party.

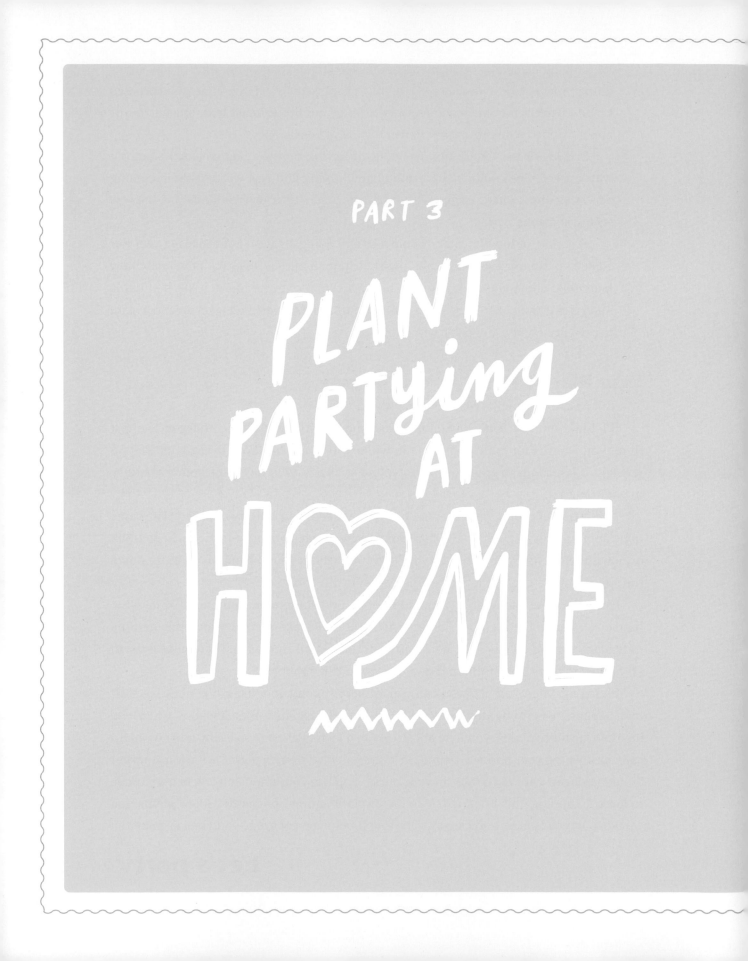

PART 3

PLANT PARTYING AT H♥ME

(where other people are unavoidable, and wearing pants is optional)

Once you begin to give more hoots about your health and happiness, it might be surprising how often you find yourself in the kitchen. Forget bars, hotels, clubs, banquet halls, Chuck E. Cheeses; the party now takes place within a five-foot radius of your fridge. When you start to care about what you put into your mouth each day, you'll realize that most restaurants aren't particularly skilled in making energy-boosting, digestion-friendly meals.

It makes sense that healthy eating would come most naturally at home. Things are easier when you have control over what comes in, what goes out, and what gets stuffed into Monica's secret closet. But becoming your own personal chef is a big role to take on, which is why this part of the book is designed to help you adjust to your new job title with ease and confidence—no need to audit community college home ec.

Learning to feel cool and collected while whipping up something that pleases both your palate *and* your body is the No. 1 thing you can (and really: *must*) do in order to take your plant party to the next level.

Here's how.

Be a Basic Bitch (or Bro)

"Basic bitch" is a horrific term for a human but a useful synonym for how you should stock your kitchen: with dime-a-dozen items that'll make knowing what to cook a cinch. The things to keep in your home are b-to-the-asic to the max.

TRENDY FOODS CAN SUCK IT

If Mother Nature could talk, she'd be LOLing at people who spend their moolah on fancy-pants products. These superfood, super trendy, super expensive, super flashy, super well-branded foods *are* like fancy pants: sparkly but unnecessary. Last I checked, regular pants still serve their purpose—they cover your tush, keep your legs warm, and allow you to go more time between shaves. While those paper-bag-waist trousers that were on fire in 2017 are just sitting in your closet, your old faithful jeans are the *goods*.

I hope you're still with me, because this is a perfect metaphor for superfood products ("fancy plants"). Healthy eating is not about the snack du jour. It's about getting to know the basics day in and day out, and treating yo'self to those fancy pants—I mean, plants—occasionally. Nobody can patent a lemon. Nobody can trademark spinach. Nobody can really profit from those basic plants, so businesses create prettily packaged, expensive products with superstar ingredients so they can make their pretty pennies. Some of those products rock; they're just not *required*.

I also want to note that eating trendy foods on top of an otherwise unhealthy diet won't do s*&t for your health. You can't go out for pepperoni pizza and eat chia pudding for dessert and call it even. As comedian Mitch Hedberg said, "That would be cool if you could eat a good food with a bad food and the good food would cover for the bad food when it got to your stomach. Like you could eat a carrot with an onion ring and they would travel down to your stomach, then they would get there, and the carrot would say, 'It's cool, he's with me.'"

That would be cool, Mitch, but truth is, eating basic most of the time is what's really cool. So when it comes to plotting the staples in your kitch, think: basic bitch. I love pumpkin spice lattes as much as the next girl from Connecticut, just without all the icky additives in your typical commercial version (recipe on page 230).

BASIC INGREDIENTS

If you don't keep healthy food in your home, you won't keep putting healthy food in your mouth. So, meet my basic bitches. I encourage you to befriend them as well. And if any of them seems intimidating, never fear—I'll be explaining the more obscure ingredients as we go.

The *s are the plants that you should try to fork up the funds for organic. The non-starred items are okay conventional, because they have a thick outer layer that blocks the chemmies from penetrating.

Basic Bitches in Your Fridge

- [at least] 1 leafy green*— kale, spinach, arugula, Swiss chard, mesclun greens

- [at least] 1 berry*—bluebs, rasps, strawbs, blacks

- [at least] 1 other fruit* you love

- [at least] 3 veggies*—bell peppers, cucumbers, zucchinis, celery, carrots, cauliflower, broccoli, Brussels sprouts, spaghetti squash, butternut squash, acorn squash, mushrooms, asparagus, tomatoes, whatever's either in season or in-style for your taste buds.

- [at least] 1 onion

- [at least] 1 sweet potato*

- [at least] 1 cooking citrus—I'm talking lemons and limes!

- [at least] 1 plant protein, like a package of tofu or a package of tempeh

- [your favorite] high-quality (and maybe gluten-free) bread, English muffins, or tortillas

- [your favorite] plant milk from almonds, rice, hemp, soy, oat, coconuts (unsweetened because you're sweet enough already)

- [at least] 1 bottle of fermented plants— kombucha, sauerkraut, or even a jar of probiotics

Basic Bitches in Your Freezer

- [at least] 2 frozen fruits*—blueberries, strawberries, mixed berries, pineapple, mango, peaches, acai
- [at least] 2 frozen veggies*—edamame, peas, broccoli, kale, spinach, asparagus, butternut squash
- [at least] 1 package of your fave veggie burgers
- Frozen bananas in a baggie (peeled)

. . . .

Frozen Plants

Some people wonder about the meaning of life and others wonder about the healthiness of frozen fruits and veggies. For the latter group, I have the answer. Frozen fruits and veggies are stellar. Those baggies are frozen at *peak* ripeness, at which time they're reached their nutritional height. Freezing locks down their nutrients like a time capsule, so you can defrost at your leisure and add to any meal like gummy vitamins without the gummy. In my book, which this is, frozen veggies are the ultimate win-win-win. They're a win because they're so nutritious. They're a win because they don't go bad in the back of your fridge, causing you to hit your face with your hand. And they're a win because they're cheap. All that to say that maybe the meaning of life *is* frozen produce?

Fermented Food

Much like Windex at Big Fat Greek Weddings, there's not much fermented foods can't do. Raw sauerkraut, kombucha, kimchi, miso, dairy-free yogurts, tempeh, and apple cider vinegar all help your digestion soar to new heights with their probiotic goodness. The more good bacteria and enzymes in our guts, the better and quicker our bodies get rid of the bad stuff, so fermented foods can speed up that whole process. This also helps with liver function, especially if it's struggling a bit after happy hour. The antibiotics we take when we get sick, as well as the Standard American Diet, wipe out the happy bacteria in our bellies, which compromises our immune system. Fermented foods helps strengthen our immunity so we can kick colds in the crotch.

. . . .

Basic Bitches for Your Pantry/Dry Goods Storage/Cabinet/Counter/Ikea Bins Under Your Bed

- Garlic

- Sea salt or pink salt

- Freshly ground black pepper

- Coconut oil, both as a spray and as an oil in a jar that is hard like butter at chilly temperatures but soft like oil at warm temperatures. The fact that butter-flavored coconut oil exists makes me shout, "What a time to be alive!" Yes, it's a more processed version of regular unadulterated coconut oil, which is why I suggest whipping it out primarily for popcorn and cupcakes.

- Extra-virgin olive oil

- [at least] 1 healthy sweetener like stevia, coconut sugar, Medjool dates, maple syrup, or raw honey. Maple syrup is mineral-rich and unprocessed, perfect in baked goods, oatmeal, dressings, sauces, granolas, and more. Stevia's my sugar-free sugar daddy for nonbaked food like cocktails, overnight oats, grapefruit, and snacks. Medjool dates are nature's candy, packed with magnesium, fiber, potassium, and iron. You'll pop 'em in smoothies, desserts, protein bars and balls, and,

of course, straight into your mouth. (Soak them in a bowl of warm water for at least ten minutes to soften them up for blending.) Coconut sugar is my 1:1 replacement for cane sugar because it has a very low glycemic index (it won't spike your blood sugar) and a nutty, rich flavor. Finally, raw honey (which is thicker than the drippy stuff found in a plastic bear) is an enzyme-rich companion for bread with nut butter, tea, or right off the spoon.

- Raw apple cider vinegar with "the mother," a fermented, packed-with-probiotics bacteria sponge. Drink a teaspoon of ACV in water to boost digestion, detoxification, and fat burning (hence my daily morning ACV drink with it on page 293), and use it in sauces, dressings, and even some baking. This one's a keeper.

- Bananas (in addition to the ones sitting pretty chilly in your freezer)

- Rolled oats (and steel-cut if you like them)

- [at least] 1 avocado, ripening on your counter (or if it's soft already, then in your fridge, oops! Move her in there!)

- [at least] 1 nut or seed*—raw almonds, walnuts, cashews, pecans, pumpkin seeds

- [at least] 2 teas (see the tea breakdown on page 265)

- [at least] 2 cans of beans*— chickpeas, black beans, pinto beans, kidney beans, lentils

- [at least] 1 grain you can boil—so basically quinoa, but a pasta made from rice, chickpeas, black beans, or lentils counts, too

- [your fave] Nut or seed butter*— almond, peanut, sunflower seed, cashew, tahini

- [your most commonly used] Ground spices. I <3 cinnamon, cayenne, nutmeg, cumin, coriander, chili powder, oregano, onion powder, garlic powder, paprika, pumpkin pie spice, cardamom, ginger, cloves, and turmeric because part of healthy cooking is starting to use seasonings to flavor the heck out of stuff. A lot of recipes out there call for a laundry list of spices, and as you get more comfortable, you'll start just adding them to food (not laundry) on your own.

- Dark chocolate bars and chips (or if you're an overachiever, the raw, unprocessed, found-in-nature form of chocolate called cacao nibs; see page 315 for the difference between the two)

- [your favorite] Hippie seeds—chia, hemp, flax

- A plant-based protein powder: If you want to lose or maintain your weight, stay mentally alert, feel calm, and not have dramatic crashes in blood sugar (which lead to cravings and binge/overeating), then you're going to want to have this around. I sneak it into everything I possibly can—blended into smoothies, whipped into yogurt, mixed in oatmeal, baked in baked goods, processed into homemade protein bars, rolled into balls, pureed into ice cream. Nearly any sweet treat provides an opportunity to add some plant-protein powder.

Sea Salt or Pink Salt

Pink's not just pretty. Those crystals might be aesthetically worthy of replacing the diamond in my engagement ring, but that's not why it's the only salt I buy. Pink or Himalayan salt is the cleanest and healthiest salt on the planet. (And, yes, it's the same NaCl used to make those Pinterest-ready lamps you see at spas and Urban Outfitters.) Himalayan salt is far superior to that regular old table salt because it's unrefined, unprocessed, mega-rich in minerals (it has over eighty-four), and helps balance our body's pH levels, which can make a big difference in our overall health. Basically, you're going to be using salt, so you might as well make it the prettiest and purest one you can.

"WOULD-BE-NICE-ABLES," A.K.A. THINGS THAT ARE AWESOME TO HAVE ON HAND AND ARE CALLED FOR IN SOME OF MY RECIPES BUT WON'T RUIN YOUR DAY IF YOU DON'T HAVE THEM AROUND:

Would-be-nice-ables in your fridge

- Coconut water

- Almond or coconut yogurt (unsweetened, plain)

- Fresh ginger root

- Hummus

- A fresh green herb* like basil, cilantro, parsley, rosemary, thyme, sage, or mint

- [your favorite] Condiments like Dijon mustard, ketchup, hot sauce

- 1 snacking citrus like grapefruit, oranges

- Shredded unsweetened coconut flakes

- A dairy-free cheese

- Miso: The 411 is that miso is a thick, salty, kinda sweet paste made from fermented soybeans. It's rich in probiotics, B vitamins, and flavor, which is why it's called for in many of my dressings, spreads, and sauces. Because it's super salty, you don't need too much to pack a punch, so a container will last you many months.

Would-be-nice-ables in your pantry/dry goods storage/cabinet/counter/space below your bed:

- Tamari, which is a gluten-free soy sauce

- Gluten-free, low-sugar granola (even better, make your own on page 263)

- Balsamic vinegar

- Nutritional yeast: "Noot yeast" is a flaky seasoning that hits all the "free's": gluten-, GMO, and dairy-free. Not only that, it tastes as close to cheese as something non-cheese can taste. You probably won't be like, "OMG, I'm eating dairy cheese right now." Its deal is more like, "Wow. I *feel* like I'm eating cheese; it's just giving me that same vibe."

  That's why noot yeast is great for sprinkling on salads and main dishes, as well as blending up to make dairy-free cheese (like the one on page 54). It's super high in vitamin B$_{12}$, and low in calories, fat, and salt, with no added sugars and preservatives. It contains all eighteen essential amino acids, which means that it's a complete protein—6 grams in 4 tablespoons.

- Cacao powder (raw chocolate powder, spelled cacAO—not cocOA)

- Mushroom powder (more on page 326)

- Veggie stock

- Vanilla extract

- Dried unsweetened fruit—like dates, mangos, papayas, figs, apricots, ginger

- Baking soda and baking powder

- [Your preferred] whole-grain baking flour, such as spelt, oat, almond flour (a.k.a. almond meal), gluten-free mix

- Canned pumpkin

- A gluten-free cracker or rice cake

Reading Between the Food Label Lines

Reading a food label can be as confusing as reading a legal document; there's a lot of mumbo jumbo to interpret. However, unlike with legal documents, you don't need to pass the bar to be able to read a bar. (Like, a snack bar.) Here's my speedy five-step process:

STEP 0: Ignore all marketing slogans. Flip right to the back of any product. The front is where the expert marketers have written their thoroughly tested big-impact BS words, and that's not for you. You're an ass-man.

STEP 1: Shoot immediately to the ingredients list.

Notice: Are there many ingredients? In processed, packaged foods, the more is *not* the merrier. You want it to be like your partner's list of ex-lovers—as short as possible. If it's over six or seven ingredients, reconsider eating it.

Next: Can you pronounce all the ingredients? It's okay if they're tough—like Hermione, Geoff, or quinoa—but do they sound like prescription drugs or things that should be in toilet bowl cleaner?

Are the first half of the ingredients *clean*? Food labels list their ingredients in order from most prominent to least so make sure that the first half are things you really want to eat.

Finally, are there any liars on the list? For example . . . did you know there are fifty-six ways to say "sugar": Agave nectar, Barbados sugar, Barley malt, Beet sugar, Blackstrap molasses, Brown rice syrup, Brown sugar, Buttered syrup, Cane juice crystals, Cane sugar, Caramel, Carob syrup, Castor sugar, Confectioners' sugar, Corn syrup, Corn syrup solids, Crystalline fructose, Date sugar, Demerara sugar, Dextran, Dextrose, Diastatic malt, Diatase, Ethyl maltol, Evaporated cane juice, Florida crystals, Fructose, Fruit juice, Fruit juice concentrate, Galactose, Glucose, Glucose solids, Golden sugar, Golden syrup, Grape sugar, High-fructose corn syrup, Honey, Icing sugar, Invert sugar, Lactose, Malt syrup, Maltose, Maple syrup, Molasses, Muscovado sugar, Organic raw sugar, Panocha, Raw sugar, Refiner's syrup, Rice syrup, Sorghum syrup, Sucrose, Sugar, Treacle, Turbinado sugar, Yellow sugar.

STEP 2: Saunter over to the "servings per."

If what you're eyeing as a single snack actually contains four servings, Houston, we have a problem. Make sure your grub is one or maybe two servings.

STEP 3: Scope out the grams of sugar.

I rarely give a food the green light if the grams of sugar is in the double digits. In general, if sugar is one of the top three to five ingredients on the label, reconsider allowing it to greet your body since sugar at the top of the list means it's the star of the show (and, again, there are *many* ways to sneak sugar in under different names).

STEP 4: Check out the fat.

If something's unusually high in fat, I take note because maybe I misinterpreted an ingredient or didn't notice how it's prepared. A perfect example is frozen sweet potato fries. They don't say "deep-fried then frozen" on the bag, *but* when their fat content is super high, I assume they were fried in lots of oil first, which means no thanks.

STEP 5: Price check.

Since healthy food often isn't the cheapest option in the store, I ask myself whether the product is worth the price. Would the store-brand equivalent be equally healthy? I double-check that I'll actually *eat it*—and I actually *want it*. Would an apple suffice? Or a bottle of water? If I want it, I get it and I don't complain about the price, 'cause I know that if I spend a little extra moolah on healthy food-la, then I'm gonna need to spend less moolah on medical crapoola moving forward.

And if you're wondering why I didn't say to look for "organic," here's my answer: Organic holds more weight with produce, and apples, pears, and berries don't typically come with a nutrition label so they're not really what I'm talking about here. Do you want to buy organic ketchup? Sure, can't hurt, but I'd rather you buy a ketchup with the highest-quality, non-processed ingredients than one with organic tomatoes and loads of cane sugar. Nah mean, amigo?

A Real Estate Lesson

I once had an organizational expert on my podcast[6] to whom I confessed sometimes ordering delivery solely because the idea of shuffling through my pan collection was too overwhelming. The lesson she taught me was, don't just keep things around because they look good. If you only use that giant stand mixer twice a year it doesn't need to be cluttering your counter when your less-sexy spiralizer could sit in its place, tempting you to make zucchini noodles weekly. Take a good hard look at which gizmos you use all the time and which you hardly use any of the time and tailor your storage solutions around that. I use coconut oil spray, liquid stevia, mushroom powder, ACV, pink salt, matcha, my waffle iron, my blender, my spiralizer, my small saucepan, and my large sauté pan at least once a day so they're all mainstays.

If Conditioner Can Be Shaving Cream . . .

Sometimes the mere idea of following a recipe can make you run right into the arms of a restaurant or your delivery app. Recipes are rad. They're helpful. This book has more than a hundred of them.

But they're not necessarily *necessary*.

You know how when you're in the shower and you realize you want to shave before you leg flirt with your hot yoga instructor? But you're out of shaving cream, so you just grab some body wash or conditioner and shave with that instead? And the world doesn't fall apart? Same goes for subbing kale for spinach. Or yellow onions for white ones. Or almond butter for peanut butter. My point is: Do your best. Use what you have. If you need to blend a smoothie with water instead of almond milk, don't have a cow. If you need to sub cane sugar for coconut sugar, sweet. If the recipe calls for two teaspoons of cinnamon, but you only have one, don't run out to the store; just make it with one.

A few other tips for recipe-less cooking:

1. **DON'T GET TOO ATTACHED.** Eventually, you won't have to follow recipes all the time. Why? Once you learn how you like your plants prepared—massaged kale, roasted sweet potatoes, sautéed onions, boiled edamame—and how to whip up a dressing or sauce by eyeballing the ingredients, making a meal will be a breeze.

6 It's the *Party in My Plants* podcast! Exactly what your ears are craving; guaranteed.

2. GET YOUR GREENS AT EVERY MEAL. Just like a margarita feels off without a lime, a meal feels *wrong* without something green. Whether it's a smoothie, a sandwich, or a side of steamed vegetables, try to make sure there's always a leafy green involved.

3. Underrated kitchen tool >>>>> YOUR EYEBALLS.

The nutrients found in fruits and veggies can be categorized by color, which makes it easy to create a balanced meal just by looking at the rainbow on your plate. You'll grow to instinctively know when your plate needs something orange or green.

. . . .

Suit Yourself

Another way to easily eat more plants (without hating or radically changing your life) is to be more like Steve Jobs, President Obama, Mark Zuckerberg, and Simon Cowell. There's a reason these powerful men make a point of wearing the same outfit every day.

Because one outfit is simply all they can afford.

Wait, scratch that. In recent years, scientists have found out that our decision-making energy is a depletable resource. "Decision fatigue" means that the more choices you make throughout a day, the more exhausted your brain becomes, and, eventually, you start leaning on laziness, impulsiveness, and what-freaking-*ever*-ness. As Obama said when he still lived in the White House: "I wear only gray or blue suits. . . . I'm trying to pare down decisions. I don't want to make decisions about what I'm eating or wearing. Because I have too many other decisions to make."

Almost everyone feels that dinner is the most difficult meal to get a handle on. Does any of this sound familiar?

◯ **"I'm great with breakfast since I have a green smoothie or oatmeal and lunch is usually a salad, but dinner is the issue."**

◯ **"Dinners are tough because my husband just wants something filling after a long day, and it's hard to be inventive and make evening meals as healthy as possible when I'm tired."**

◯ **"I'm completely fried after a long day, which means I unfortunately usually eat something unhealthy like fries."**

Remember: The more choices you make, the more exhausted your brain becomes, and, eventually, your decisions fall back on laziness, impulsiveness, and "what-freaking-*ever*" ness. The goal with healthy eating is to eat well all day long, not just, like, until it's dark and your brain is kaput and you order pizza. The way you make your brain not kaput is by not expending so much freaking energy on your food.

Take advantage of mix-'n'-matching. I rotate through three breakfasts, six snacks, two lunches, eight dinners, and two desserts each week. Look at what you ate today and consider: How can you vary your plants while keeping a familiar foundation so you don't waste any brainpower? If you started your day with oatmeal with blueberries, what if tomorrow you added banana and a dollop of peanut butter instead? And the day after that you went tropical with chopped pineapple and coconut? And then you went dessert-for-breakfast, 'cuz it's FRIYAY, and mixed in cacao nibs and almond butter? And then you went superfood-buck-wild and added chia seeds and goji berries? And you wrapped up the week with apple-pie oatmeal: apple, cinnamon, raw walnuts, and raisins?

Some Kitchen Tools That Will Make Kitchen Life Much More Bitchin':

A salad spinner

Think of a salad spinner like a hair dryer: Your hair can dry without one, but it'll take longer, and get your shoulders wet. A salad spinner takes the wet washed greens and whips them around fast to centrifuge the water, making them perfectly dry and clean. (Nice if you don't like eating a salad bowl full of wet, soggy lettuce!)

A steamer basket

You'll want a steamer basket, which is a ridiculously cheap piece of kitchen equipment that I liken to a loofah—the opposite of hip, but highly underrated. To use a steamer basket, expand it in a pot. Add water but only enough so it's just about coming through the basket. Turn the stove onto high heat, cover the pot, and once you hear the water boiling and you see steam wafting up through the holes in the steamer basket, add your veggie, secure the lid, and let the steam do its work.

A food processor

Having a food processor in addition to a blender is a luxury, perhaps, but one that'll make life so much easier. Like your car having heated seats in the winter, your workout top having thumbholes, or your feet having rain boots in the rain. The absence of those things won't kill ya, but doesn't their presence make your life better, easier, and more comfortable? Such is the story with a food processor. What differentiates a food processor from a blender is the blade. A processor's blade is designed for chopping, a blender's blade is designed for . . . blending. Each excels at things the other struggles with. For example, a food processor can chop up perfect salsa, while a blender will make your salsa a gazpacho. A food processor can chop up your nuts for granola, while a blender will turn your nuts into dust. (They can both puree for creamy soup, banana ice cream, or smooth sauce.) Basically, blenders need liquid to get the job done; a food processor doesn't. If you're just making food for yourself, or yourself +1, a small processor will be all you need.

A spiralizer

A spiralizer is a weird device both in look and sound. IT IS WEIRD. IT'S REALLY, REALLY WEIRD. But I encourage you not to resist. The spiralizer was born to help create those garnishes that are typically seen on Asian dishes in restaurants. I guess somewhere along the way, someone decided that veggie noodles were a waistline-friendly way to replace a bowl of carb-filled pasta, and so the zoodle (zucchini noodle) was created. Since then, innovative eaters have learned to spiralize sweet potatoes into swoodles, butternut squash into boodles, bell peppers into poodles, and apples into . . . apple pasta!

What's with All the Glass Jars?

It's hard to find a Pinterest smoothie that's *not* in a mason jar. Look: Glass jars are awesome. They feel enchanting on your lips, they have a nice heft to them, cleaning them is a breeze, they're environmentally friendly, they don't leak plastic chemical crap into your non-crap food, and they cost little to nothing (an old nut butter jar makes a perfect smoothie cup). They also make great overnight oats containers, are wonderful for storing leftover soups and sauces, and are lovely all-around glassware. And cocktail glasses. Bottom line: Save your pickle jars!

What About Protein?

Elephant in the room. Steak on the plate. Gorilla (who eats a plant-based diet, FYI) in the jungle. I want to address the protein thang right up top because I'm as sick of hearing "Where do you get your protein?" as Rachel is about hearing Ross say, "We were on a break." In this case, the protein thing has a definite right answer.

When I first started eating primarily plants back in the day (as in when Netflix was still a mail-order DVD rental service), the main rebuttal I had for those cliché jokes/condescending questions/genuine concern was basically "Leave me alone!" Fast-forward four years and I had upped my exercise from spinning and hot yoga to Insanity/P90X/CrossFit–type stuff and I found myself getting colds after workouts and *not* getting the toned muscles that lifting weights promised me. My now husband, then new boyfriend, a then big meat eater, now big plant-eater, would look at my dinners of brown rice pasta with pesto and veggies and ask, "Uhh, darling, where's the protein?" and I'd snap back that "I get enough protein from plants" and eat a whole avocado to try to get full. It's no wonder my body was squishy, not swole. No wonder I was always hungry.

Eventually I bought a bag of brown rice plant protein like the buff guys at my gym. It was straight out of an infomercial. I added that protein to my smoothie and was like "Golly! There *is* a better way!" because I felt full and satisfied for hours. Then I started adding beans or tofu or tempeh to my meals and that fab extra flab started to fade away like those Netflix DVDs.

It turns out that the whole "enough protein from plants" rebuttal only works if you work it. Your goal, from here on out, is to intentionally add protein to every meal. Bonus points if you can add it to every snack, too.

Protein, by the way, isn't just clutch because you lift heavy things or because you're fearmongered about its importance. Protein is what fills you up! As in, no mas shoveling an entire bag of popcorn in your mouth at three because you're still ravenous after lunch. In the same vein, protein is what helps to alleviate those unpleasant blood sugar roller-coaster rides, which can prevent the scientific condition known as HANGER. Protein helps your body build and repair tissues, bones, muscles, cartilage, skin, and blood; make cool chemicals like hormones and enzymes; and keep your immunity, heart, and respiratory systems strong AF.

Your goal, from here on out, is to intentionally add protein to every meal.

Here's what's sick about getting your protein from plants: It gives you all the above benefits without also giving you high cholesterol, clogging your arteries, or turning your body into an acidic disease-developing machine.

This is pretty exciting stuff for plant protein. And for you.

Here are my favorite plant proteins to party with:

- Tofu, 10 grams of protein per ½ cup

- Tempeh, 16 grams of protein per ½ cup

- Edamame, 17 grams of protein per cup

- Lentils, 18 grams of protein per 1 cup, cooked

- Beans, 15 grams of protein per 1 cup, cooked

- Peas, 9 grams of protein per 1 cup

- Chickpea and lentil pastas, 14 grams per 2 ounces

- Brown rice protein powder, 18 grams of protein per ¼ cup (which is usually 1 scoop)

- Quinoa, 8-ish grams of protein per ½ cup, cooked

- Chia and flaxseeds, 4 to 5 grams of protein per 2 tablespoons

- Oats, 5.5 grams of protein per ½ cup

- Hemp seeds, 10 grams of protein per 2 to 3 tablespoons

- Nutritional yeast, 12 grams of protein per 3 tablespoons

- Teff, 5 grams of protein per ½ cup

- Seeds (sunflower, sesame, pumpkin) and nuts (raw almonds, walnuts, cashews, pistachios), 7 to 9 grams of protein per ¼ cup

- Sprouted bread and tortillas, 4 to 6 grams of protein per slice/wrap

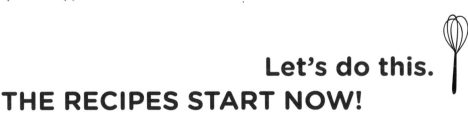

Let's do this.
THE RECIPES START NOW!

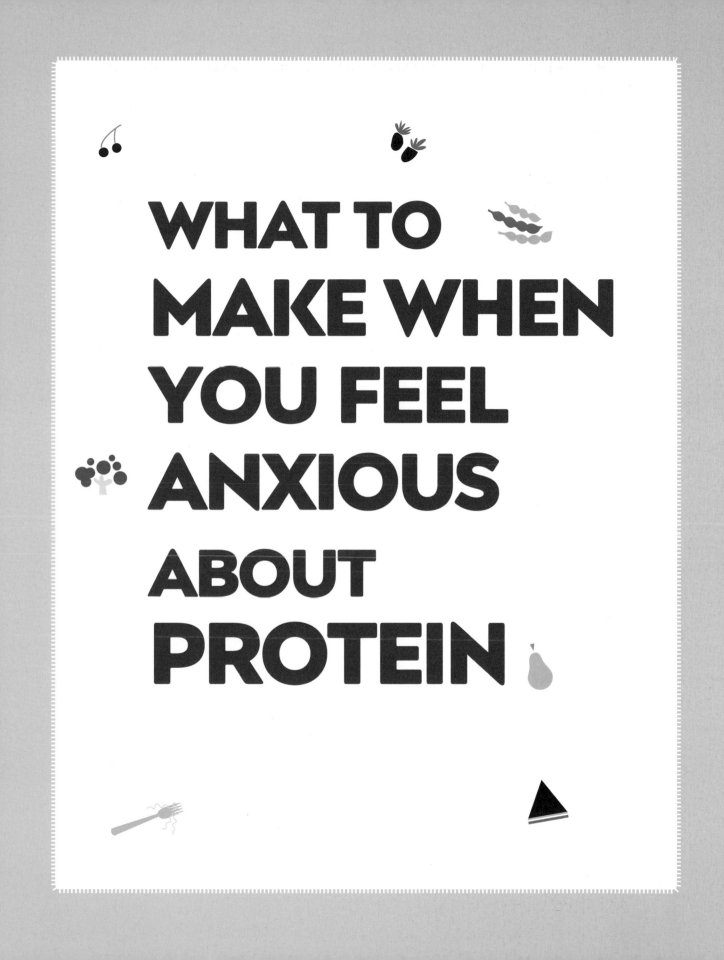

WHAT TO MAKE WHEN YOU FEEL ANXIOUS ABOUT PROTEIN

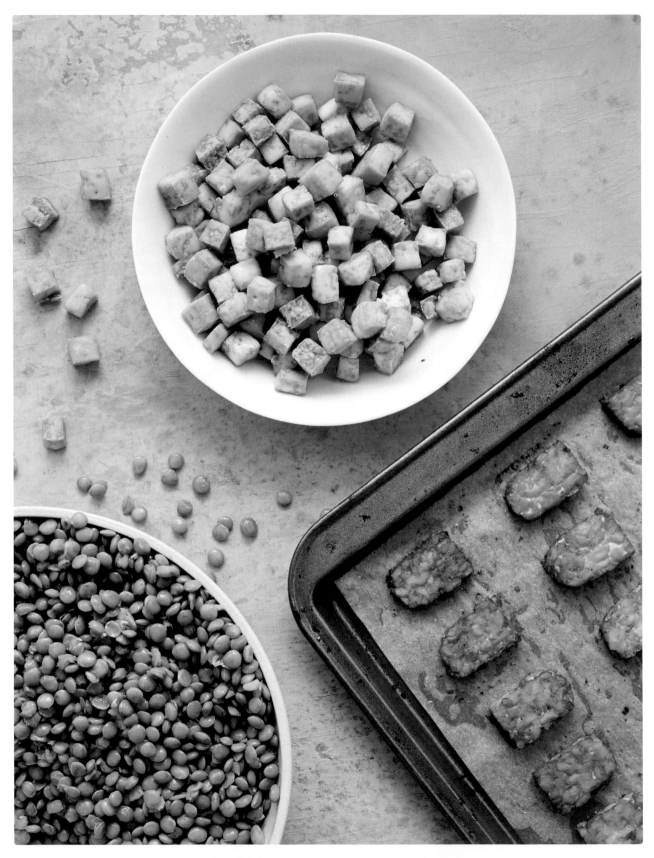

From left to right: cooked lentils, Camo Tofu, TGIT

TGIT

(Thank God It's Tempeh—that's actually good)

Tempeh is freaky. It looks like it'd be a better fit as a prop in *Stranger Things* than a thing you put in your mouth. But once you get through the mental barrier—and trust me, I wouldn't put anything in this book that I don't *know* will rock your world—you're going to really be into this versatile protein. Tempeh is a patty made from split and fermented soybeans, which is bound together by enzymes, which make it easy to digest and great for gut health. Tempeh's its best self with some oil/vinegar marinade, because it takes on whatever flavor it's soaked in. This is my go-to basic recipe that can you can add to virtually every savory dish that needs a protein bump.

SERVES 2 TO 4

1 tablespoon olive oil

1 tablespoon tamari

1 tablespoon ACV (apple cider vinegar)

½ tablespoon maple syrup

⅛ to ¼ teaspoon black pepper

½ teaspoon garlic powder

1 8-ounce package tempeh (I prefer the brand Lightlife and its "original" variety)

1. Preheat the oven to 375°F. Line a baking sheet with parchment paper.
2. Whisk the olive oil, tamari, ACV, maple syrup, black pepper, and garlic powder together in a big bowl.
3. Remove the tempeh from the package and cut it in half the long way. Then cut those halves into roughly ¼-inch slices.
4. Take the pieces of tempeh and coat them fully in the marinade that you whisked in the bowl.
5. Add the coated tempeh to the prepared baking sheet. Spread it out on the baking sheet.
6. Bake it for 10 minutes, flip it around to cook the opposite side of each piece, and bake for another 5 to 8 minutes.
7. Let cool and add to whatever for a hefty dose of protein.

NOTE: Even though it wasn't my intention, my recipe testers claimed this tasted like chicken. One said it was a perfect meat substitute in any dish and another told me she dipped it in ketchup like chicken nuggets and flashed back to her childhood. The more you know.

Camo Tofu

Meet an easy camouflage-able, add-to-anything baked/roasted tofu, a.k.a.: what to make when you don't know how to make good tofu or you don't love tofu but really want to. It's called "Camo Tofu" because its purpose is to act like a chameleon that gives any dish a protein boost without having to think too hard about it. Add it to pizza, pasta, noodles, rice, salad, sandwiches, wraps, tacos, fajitas, quesadillas, burritos, stir-fries, pad Thai, quinoa, soups, stews, even take-out dishes. It's slightly crunchy on the outside and sensually soft on the inside.

In my tofu recipes you'll see "press tofu" as one of your duties. This means to remove your slab of tofu from the package and place it sandwiched between two cutting boards, right by the sink so the liquid that gets pressed out from the tofu drains into the sink. Place something heavy on top of the top cutting board—I love to use stacks of cookbooks! Every couple of minutes, tilt the whole cutting board + books + tofu sandwich so the liquid getting pressed out of the tofu pours into the sink. Ideally, you want to do this for about a half hour but don't stress if you only have ten minutes—or the time it takes for your oven to heat up!

SERVES 2 TO 4

1 package firm or extra-firm tofu (non-GMO and organic)

1 tablespoon extra-virgin olive oil

¼ teaspoon sea salt or pink salt

1. Preheat the oven to 400°F. Line a baking sheet with parchment paper.
2. If time allows, press the tofu; 20 minutes is swell, 1 hour is super!
3. Cut the tofu into cubes, the smaller the better.
4. Throw the tofu cubes into a mixing bowl and add the olive oil and salt and toss the tofu around so it gets coated as evenly as possible. Feel free to sprinkle on other spices you have and love (like garlic powder, onion powder, freshly ground black pepper, or chili powder).
5. Spread the tofu on the prepared baking sheet and bake for 25 minutes. Shuffle the tofu around about halfway through to help it cook more evenly.
6. Let cool and add to everything. Store leftovers sealed in the fridge.

AFTER [PARTY] THOUGHT:

This is a bomb "when you make any make many" (page 100) recipe. Might as well double or triple it so you can throw camo tofu into whatever throughout the week.

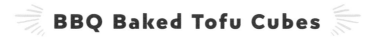

BBQ Baked Tofu Cubes

Two ingredients that comprise one of the easiest ways to get your plant protein. These cubes are great stuffed in baked sweet potatoes, quinoa, and veggie dishes, on salads and pasta or zucchini noodles with pesto, in wraps and tacos, and popped right into your mouth. I guarantee you'll never look at a naked block of tofu helplessly again.

SERVES 2 TO 4

1 package of firm tofu (non-GMO and organic)

⅓ cup of your fave BBQ sauce

1. Press the tofu for as much as time allows; 20 minutes is swell, 1 hour is super!
2. In the meantime, preheat the oven to 400°F. Line a baking sheet with parchment paper.
3. Cut the tofu into small chunks. The smaller, the crispier they'll come out.
4. Place the tofu chunks in a medium bowl and cover them with the BBQ sauce. Mix well so the sauce covers all of the tofu chunks.
5. Add the tofu to the prepared baking sheet.
6. Bake for 15 minutes.
7. After 15 minutes, pop open the oven and move the tofu chunks around so they cook evenly.
8. Bake for another 15 minutes.
9. Remove and enjoy. Store leftovers sealed in the fridge.

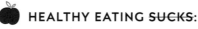 **HEALTHY EATING ~~SUCKS~~:**

"WOW, they are addicting! I honestly was expecting this to be really boring and bland because plain tofu is not my jam; however, the slight saltiness and chewy texture made for an addicting protein-filled snack." —**ML**

 NOTE: Look for a bottle that contains the lowest grams of sugar you can find. Primal Kitchen (with 2 grams of sugar per serving) rocks, followed by Woodstock Farms and Annie's, whose 7 grams of sugar per serving is from organic cane sugar, and Organicville, from organic agave.

Sweet-Ass Sriracha Tofu

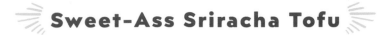

Another sweet and spicy way to make tofu tasty.

SERVES 2 TO 4

1 package firm or extra-firm tofu (non-GMO and organic)

2 tablespoons sriracha

2 tablespoons tamari

1½ teaspoons honey or maple syrup

1. Preheat the oven to 400°F. Line a baking sheet with parchment paper.
2. Press the tofu for as much as time allows; 20 minutes is swell, 1 hour is super!
3. While the tofu is being pressed, mix together the sriracha, tamari, and honey in a small bowl. Set aside.
4. Cut the tofu into small chunks. The smaller, the crispier they'll come out.
5. Add the tofu to a medium bowl and cover with the sriracha mixture. Mix well so the sauce covers all the tofu chunks.
6. Add the tofu to the prepared baking sheet.
7. Bake for 15 minutes.
8. After 15 minutes, move the tofu chunks around so they cook evenly.
9. Bake for another 15 minutes.
10. Remove and add to whatever.
11. Store leftovers sealed in the fridge.

WHAT TO MAKE WHEN YOU CRAVE CHEESE

I am well aware that dairy might play a leading role in many of your favorite food. Much like Robert De Niro, it's in nearly everything. But much like Robert De Niro's not-so-favorite son-in-law, dairy really is a focker. It's been scientifically linked to acne, cancer, and weight gain as well as stomachaches, poop problems, gas, and bloating. So if you're suffering from any of the above, it's time to mooooooo-ve right along.

I'm not saying you won't occasionally get nostalgic for an Oreo McFlurry, but I am saying that you will feel so good that they'll become a fondish memory.

EASY DAIRY SWAPS

There ain't nothing as creamy and dreamy as dairy. *Or is there?*

How about instead of whole milk in your coffee you try coconut milk? Instead of thickening your soups with cream, reach for that can of coconut milk, too. Consider coconut or almond milk yogurt in granola. Smear almond or peanut butter on your bagel instead of cream cheese, and hummus on your sandwich instead of mayo. Enhance a baked sweet potato with butter-flavored coconut oil or tahini instead of butter or sour cream, and thicken sauces with pureed cashews instead of cream. Load guacamole into your burrito instead of queso and sour cream, and pile veggies onto your pizza or pasta instead of cheese. Instead of ice cream with cow's milk, make soft serve with bananas. What if you baked with coconut oil rather than butter? And almond milk instead of skim? Blend a hemp- or rice-based protein powder into your smoothies instead of whey. Crudité's better with hummus than with ranch dip, popcorn's better with coconut oil than doused in butter, and dark chocolate whoops milk chocolate's booty.

All the above are easy-peasy swaps, but there's one thing that you might notice is missing: cheese.

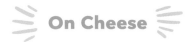

As I mentioned, back when I used to perform stand-up, I had a joke about people telling me, "I could never live without cheese." I'd go, "Really? Pretty sure you could. Pretty sure you couldn't live after getting hit by a truck or falling off a cliff, but a mozzarella stick deficiency? Not likely a cause of death."

I didn't say it was a great bit. But because I believed that this whole thing was bogus, I delivered it with so much conviction that everyone LOLed.

I was cheerfully cheese-free for ten years. But then, four years ago, in Greece, I tried soft goat cheese. And feta. And pecorino, which is Parmesan's sheep cheese doppelgänger. And soon I became the butt of my own joke. Because quite frankly, I now could *never* live without cheese.

But here's how I healthfully live with it.

1. Cheese is not a staple ingredient. Cheese is a once-in-a-while treat to make other things taste super good. My vote is that every so often you can gleefully savor the experience of adding a dairy delight to a dish. But cheese is a garnish—not a base. And it's a once-in-a-while treat, like a face mask, not a staple, like a face wash.

2. Cheese quality matters. A lot. The most. I am more attentive to the quality of my occasional cheese treat than I am to spelling errors on birthday cards. And this means no cow cheese. It's just too pumped with antibiotics and lord knows what else (having to do with our country's messed-up industrial farm system) for my body to break down, which is a big part of what leads to the bummer side effects of dairy we talked about earlier. But I don't have a cow about it! Instead, I go for the goat. And the sheep.

Goat milk is easier on our bods than cow's milk: It's lower in lactose, for one, which makes it easier for us to digest. Lactose, the sugar found in dairy, is part of what makes dairy so yucky for our bodies to begin with, so choosing a lower-lactose alternative will be gentler on your digestion and less likely to cause allergic reactions like skin issues.

Casein, which is a protein found in milk from cows, goats, and sheep, is another reason so many of us are dairy intolerant. But not all casein is the same. When we react negatively (IBS, gastrointestinal struggles, acne, eczema) to dairy, it's A1 beta-casein that we're sensitive to, which is found in milk produced by the majority of dairy cows in the United States, Western Europe, and Australia. Goat milk, on the other hand, contains A2 beta-casein, which is less inflammatory and less likely to cause an intolerance. (In fact, the chemical composition of goat milk makes it similar to human breast milk, which is why some cultures wean their babies by giving them goat milk.)

Also, since goat milk is more popular in other countries, 50 percent of the goat cheese products consumed in the United States are imported from France, which has stricter food regulations. And the goat and sheep milk industry here ain't as effed up as the cow milk industry. Goats and sheep aren't pumped with steroids and antibiotics the way cows are.

So when I do buy cheese, it's only made from goat milk or sheep milk. And when I'm out and about, I ask which lactating animal it comes from. Which sometimes means the server has to ask the chef. And then the chef has to get her package of the cheese and read the label. Because here's a not-fun fact about feta: It's often phony. A lot of feta served in restaurants in the United States is actually a "feta-style" cheese—from cow's milk. If I ask and find out that the feta cheese comes from cow, not goat or sheep, I not-so-sheepishly say *no, thanks.*

3. Cut the cheese. I avoided all dairy for ten years. It was rad! I got thrust into the dairy-less life while working my first job at Cold Stone Creamery. Let me rephrase: While working my *dream job* at Cold Stone Creamery. Singing parody songs while serving people the one thing in the world that's impossible to not smile at while receiving. While stuffing my face with all-I-could-eat ice cream and waffle cones before we got customers at 10:30 a.m. and during lulls throughout the day.

Until that time I realized I'd made myself lactose intolerant. Dear reader: I almost pooped in my pants.

The long story short is that I was on antibiotics. This was years before Gwyneth Gooped about probiotics, so unbeknownst to me, for two weeks I had been depleting my stomach of any helpful microbes while still filling up on gallons of ice cream. It came to a head while I was driving around with a friend of mine. I squeezed my cheeks and prayed while rocking out to Gnarls Barkley's mega-hit "Crazy." Which was both popular and appropriate at the time.

After the near-poopcident, I got a restraining order on all cheese, milk, cream, butter, or ice cream that came from an animal, and that, coupled with my plant-based revelation four years later, changed my body and life and yada yada yada.

But then, on a whim, I tried that goat cheese. It was in a salad I really wanted and I didn't want to try to say "no cheese please" in Greek because I had seen the owner throw a plate a few minutes prior, which I know was to celebrate, but still it was scary. I waited. I didn't feel sick. I actually felt good. Years before, listening to my body meant cutting out all dairy; now, it meant taking baby steps back to a sometimes relationship with it.

Some of us digest dairy better than others. Pay attention to any negative effects of eating even high-quality dairy, like skin issues, digestive distress, and congestion. If you're not sure, cut it out completely for two to three weeks and then reintroduce it slowly. If you feel the same, your skin's the same, then you're good to go. If you look and feel different, you'll be incentivized to lay low.

4. Don't fake it; make it. When people decide to ditch dairy, they tend to switch to processed "fake cheeses" and sugary pints of dairy-free ice cream. Switching from loads of dairy to loads of crap food is about as good for your body as switching from regular cigarettes to regular cigars. Instead, make a substitute with real ingredients that'll help you get past those creamy cravings.

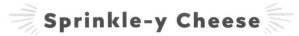

Sprinkle-y Cheese

A jar of sprinkle-y cheese lives on my counter at all times because at all times I find myself eating things that would taste better with sprinkle-y cheese. It's Parmesan-y and nonperishable, and, like peanut butter, dangerous with a spoon nearby.

MAKES ABOUT 1 CUP

¾ cup raw cashews, pumpkin seeds, pecans, or walnuts

2 tablespoons nutritional yeast

¼ teaspoon pink salt or sea salt

1. Preheat the oven to 300°F.

2. Spread the nuts on a clean rimmed baking sheet and toast for 6 to 10 minutes. You'll know they're done when they're deliciously fragrant and lightly golden.

3. Process the toasted nuts or seeds in your food processor until they're like coarse sand. Not Caribbean sand, East Coast sand.

4. Add the nutritional yeast and salt to the food processor and process until it's your desired texture.

5. Sprinkle on salads or pasta dishes, into wraps, or on steamed or roasted veggies.

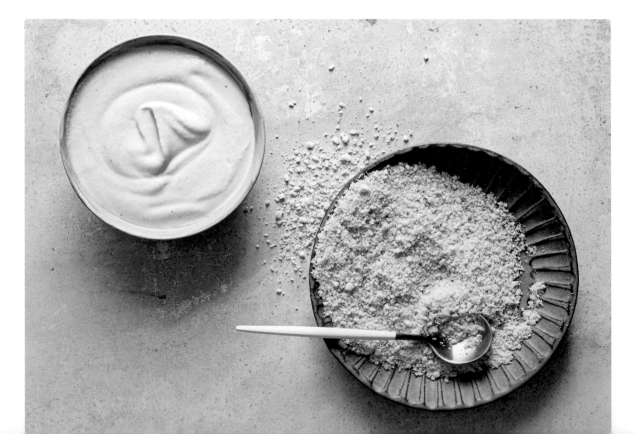

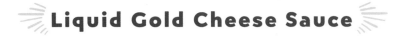

Liquid Gold Cheese Sauce

Reminiscent in texture and color to Velveeta (the "liquid gold" that my mom discovered was the orange ticket that got me to eat boiled broccoli), this cheese sauce could be the orange ticket to get you to say bye to Velveeta. It makes all vegetables taste better, works on mac and cheese, and gets smothered all over Nacho-Unhealthy Nachos (page 193).

MAKES ABOUT 1 CUP

1½ cups cashews (ideally presoaked with warm water for 1 to 4 hours if you can swing it)

3 tablespoons freshly squeezed lemon juice (1 to 2 lemons)

1 teaspoon sea salt

¼ cup nutritional yeast

1 garlic clove

½ teaspoon chili powder

½ teaspoon Dijon mustard

Pinch of turmeric (optional)

1. Drain and rinse the cashews if you soaked them and add the lemon juice, ¾ cup water, the salt, nutritional yeast, garlic, chili powder, mustard, and turmeric, if using, to your blender.
2. Blend until wildly creamy and use the opposite of sparingly.
3. Store leftovers sealed in your refrigerator.

True Life: I Got Cheeseburger Cheated On

I will never forget the moment that my college boyfriend Andrew muttered those seven magical words: "I haven't been completely honest with you."

Naturally, my mind immediately went to "Who the hell is she?!" But before I could ask, Andrew added, "I've been sneaking burgers behind your back."

It turns out, she was a Big Mac. With cheese. And probably bacon.

I was stunned.

MY BOYFRIEND WAS HAVING A FAST-FOOD AFFAIR!

A flank fling!

He'd been committing meat-dultery!

I wish I could tell you I had a sense of humor about it, but I felt like the rug had been pulled out from under me. *Is this why I see him park outside our apartment and not come in for ten minutes? Is he downing chicken nuggets? When he's in the bathroom with the door locked, is he bingeing on jerky?*

It felt as devastating as a real affair. I was confused and betrayed. I thought we were equally in love with Sunday morning tofu scrambles and buckwheat blueberry flaxseed pancakes. How could I have been so blind?

Turns out, I wasn't blind. I was the food police, which is a recipe for disaster in any relationship. Back in the day, I wasn't just on plant patrol for my boyfriend; I would make my parents feel terrible, I'd shame my sister, and I'd guilt my besties about their diets. I didn't mean to hurt the people I loved. I was "taking care of them," I told myself. I was too blinded by my desire to help my peeps eat healthy food to realize that I was making them resent that healthy food, and resent me. (Andrew was also a conflict-averse dude who'd rather sneak a burger than say, "I know you're happily sailing along on your plant boat, but my ticket is for the meat train, so I'd like to have a chicken sandwich now and then.")

Andrew is now married to a lady I can only imagine makes a mean meatloaf.

That breakup changed me. It taught me how to chill so Jesse doesn't have to sweat ordering a sirloin. Because I learned from my mistakes, my current relationship is a generally healthy one (both when it comes to food and otherwise). When I met my hubby, the only vegetable in his life was ketchup. Well, honestly, the only thing in his fridge was ketchup. Which makes it all the more interesting that six years later we're in a place where he's saying, "Are you sure I should get the burger?" and I'm saying, "Yeah, c'mon, just do it!" More on that in a bit, but first, lemme roll out my seven tricks for not letting tofu come between true love, which also means your relationship with your siblings, your friends, your parents, your kids, your co-workers, or your piano teacher.

The Art of His + Her + Their Meals

His and her meals are simple but worth explaining. All you do is make one base with different protein options to please all parties. For me, that often means making myself roasted Camo Tofu (page 48) while Jesse makes roasted chicken. It could be cooking a pot of lentils while your other half sautés ground turkey. Because I only cook plants, my lover is left to his own devices if he wants a nonplant protein. But maybe you're able and willing to make your family their preferred meals, in which case you're an angel and you can tell the benefactors of your angelic ways that this girl Talia says they're in charge of washing every single dish.

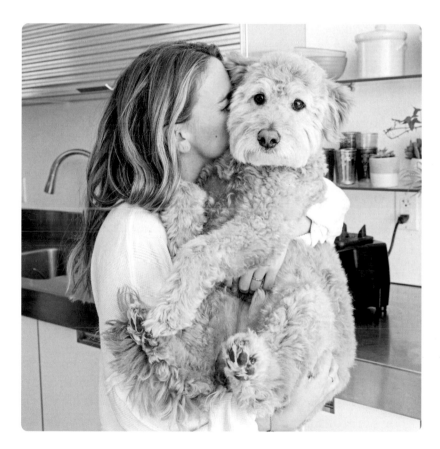

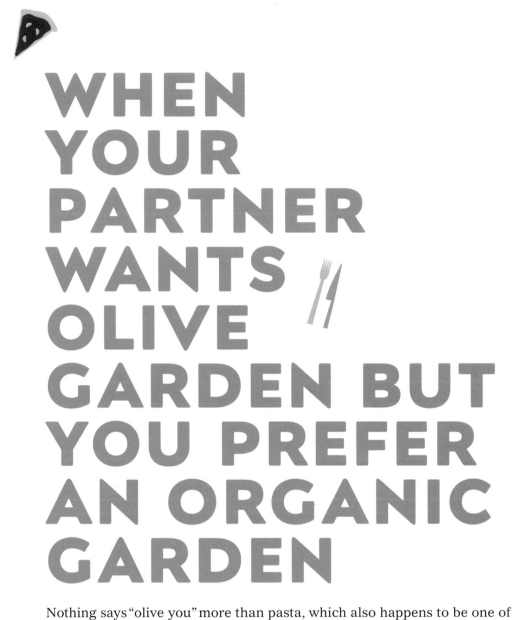

WHEN YOUR PARTNER WANTS OLIVE GARDEN BUT YOU PREFER AN ORGANIC GARDEN

Nothing says "olive you" more than pasta, which also happens to be one of the easiest dishes to make into his and hers. Choose your own adventure when it comes to protein, and these dinners will please both of your palates.

Penne Alllmost Vodka with Beats Meat Balls

Out of all my recipes here, this pasta gets that universal cooking show audible "mm-mmm" the most frequently—and most passionately. I also hear, "I can't believe it's not dairy!" like we're in a real-life infomercial. The mushroom-lentil meatballs are not required but are awe-inspiring.

SERVES 4

Beats Meat Balls (page 62)

FOR THE SAUCE

1 cup store-bought marinara/tomato sauce

½ cup raw cashews

½ teaspoon sea salt

2 teaspoons coconut sugar

½ cup packed fresh basil, plus more for garnish

FOR THE REST OF THE DISH

1 package of your fave pasta, like chickpea pasta, zoodles, brown rice pasta, lentil pasta, or a combo

2 to 3 cups chopped kale or spinach

1 to 2 cups chopped cherry tomatoes (optional)

Pinch of sea salt

Coconut or olive oil

1. Make your Beats Meat Balls.

2. When you get to baking the balls, start your Penne Alllmost Vodka sauce by blending the marinara, cashews, salt, coconut sugar, and basil until, well, super saucy.

3. Set that aside and cook the pasta per the instructions on the package.

4. Sauté the kale and cherry tomatoes with a pinch of sea salt and a spray or drizzle of coconut oil.

5. Heat up your sauce in a saucepan over low heat. You want it warm like the pasta and veggies, but be careful not to burn it.

6. At this point, your Beats Meat Balls should be done, so remove them from the oven.

continued

HEALTHY EATING ~~SUCKS~~:

"My boyfriend, who has not completely transformed his diet, said, 'Can we have this every night?' " **—JV**

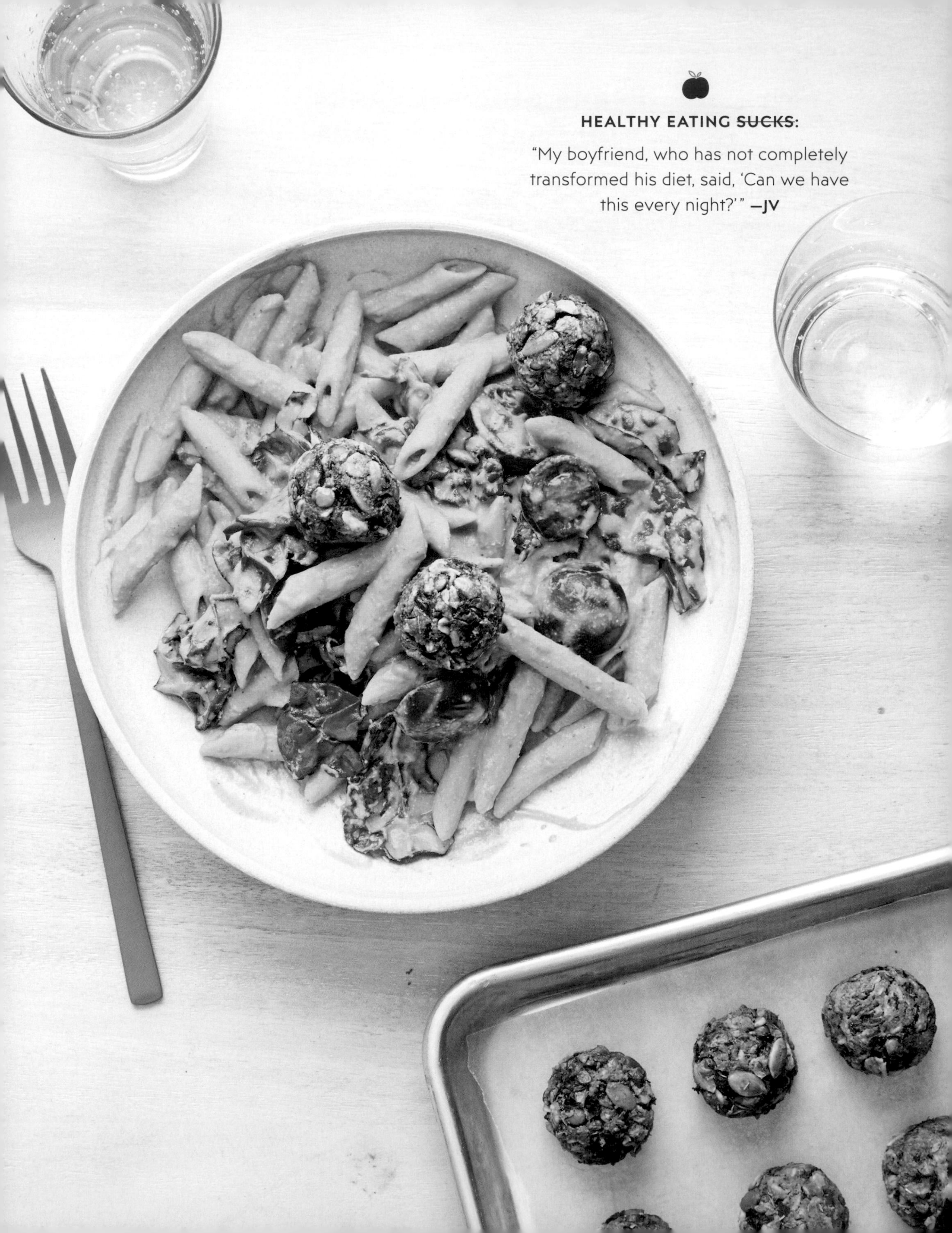

7. When everything's cooked to perfection, combine it all together for even *more* perfection.

8. Serve sprinkled with basil.

NOTE: Read the sauce label like you're reading and rereading your flight itinerary before pressing "purchase!" If you see "sugar" or "cheese" listed in the ingredients, shout "Mayday!," or just get another jar.

Beats Meat Balls
(Mushroom-Lentil Balls)

MAKES ABOUT 20 BALLS

1 cup dry green lentils

1 tablespoon ground flaxseed

2 cups chopped mushrooms (I use button mushrooms, but cremini would be delicious, too)

2 cups chopped kale or spinach, or a blend

1½ teaspoons coconut or olive oil

1 cup gluten-free oats

½ cup almond flour (if you have a nut allergy, sub ½ cup oats for the almond flour, or use a different flour)

¼ cup raw pumpkin or sunflower seeds

½ cup fresh chopped basil (optional)

1 teaspoon pink salt or sea salt

1 teaspoon dried oregano

½ teaspoon garlic powder

2 teaspoons smoked paprika

1. Add the lentils plus 2 cups water to a pot, cover, and bring to a boil. Remove the lid, reduce the heat, and simmer until all of the water has vanished.

2. Mix the flaxseed and 3 tablespoons water in a small dish or cup. Set aside. Sauté the mushrooms and kale with the coconut oil in a pan over high heat for about 5 minutes, until soft. Set aside. I like to add a pinch of salt while sautéing.

3. Preheat the oven to 350°F.

4. Once your lentils are soft, mash them with a potato masher or a fork, leaving some whole pieces for texture, then add to a large bowl.

5. Add your mushroom/greens mix to the bowl. Add the flax egg, oats, almond flour, pumpkin seeds, and fresh basil (if using). Mix well.

6. Add the salt, oregano, garlic powder, and paprika. Taste it and add more flava if you want.

7. Allow the dough to set for 3 to 5 minutes so the oats soak up some liquid.

8. Shape into heaping tablespoon–size balls and place on a rimmed baking sheet lined with parchment paper.

9. Bake these baller balls for 25 to 30 minutes, or until they're browned and feel a little crispy to the touch.

10. Store leftovers covered in the fridge.

 LEFTOVERS ARE THE BESTOVERS:

Leftover balls are excellent heated up in a toaster oven. They're also delectable cold on salads, and in other pasta dishes like the Avocadodisiac Creamy Pasta (page 77).

AFTER [PARTY] THOUGHT:

Freeze some of the Beats Meat Balls batter before rolling them into balls. On a lazy night, let that thaw, roll into balls, and easily bake from there.

HEALTHY EATING SUCKS:

"I left these out after making them because I had to run some errands When I came home, my real-meat-loving boyfriend had finished half of them." **—RA**

Smooth as Butter[Nut Squash] Creamy Pasta Bake

This is one of those "if you've got it, flaunt it" kinds of recipes, instead of one of those "hair extensions" kinds. Rather than try to punk you into thinking you're eating Kraft when you're clearly wearing a clip-on, this embraces the smooth and creamy gift from the ground that is butternut squash and makes you feel appreciation for that expensive-but-worth-it thing called a high-speed blender. If you also appreciate your fingertips and want to keep them, consider buying pre-peeled and chopped butternut squash.

MAKES 4 OR 5 GENEROUS SERVINGS

DISH

16 ounces dry pasta shells

1 tablespoon olive oil

½ medium yellow onion, chopped

½ teaspoon sea salt or pink salt, plus more as needed

3 garlic cloves, chopped

2 cups vegetable broth

4 cups peeled, diced butternut squash (about half a medium squash)

1 tablespoon tamari

1 teaspoon Dijon mustard

½ teaspoon paprika (smoked or sweet)

⅛ teaspoon freshly ground black pepper

½ cup unsweetened plain almond milk

1 tablespoon freshly squeezed lemon juice (about half a lemon)

1 tablespoon nutritional yeast

TOPPING

½ cup almond meal

1 teaspoon dried thyme

½ teaspoon smoked paprika

2 tablespoons nutritional yeast

½ teaspoon sea salt or pink salt

1 tablespoon olive oil

HEALTHY EATING ~~SUCKS~~:

"My boyfriend was so skeptical, but once he took a bite he wanted a whole serving!" **—HBS**

"I am not kidding you. I think I could eat this for every meal." **—CA**

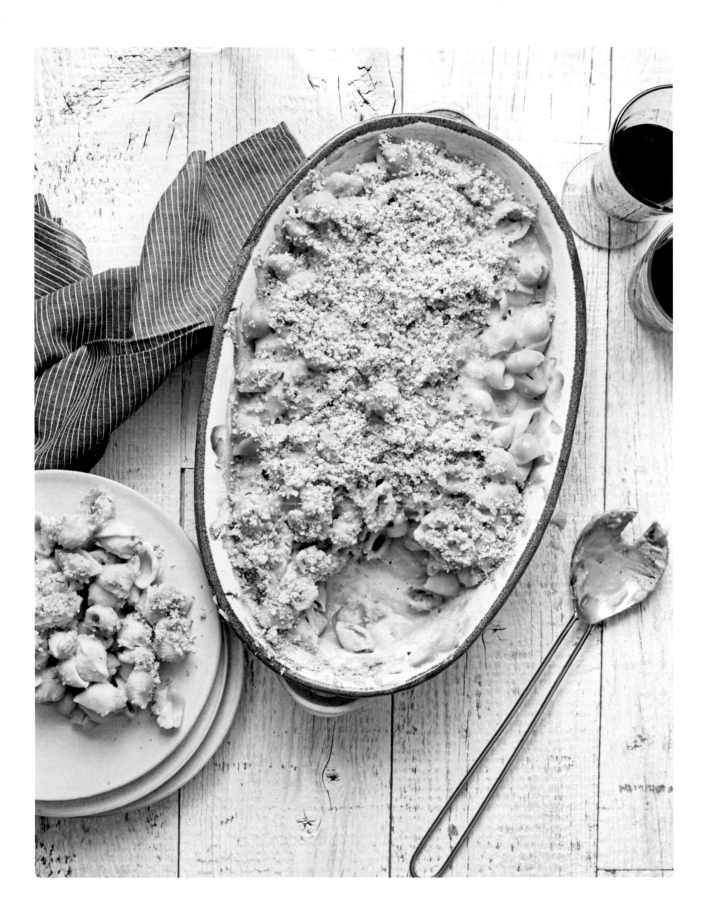

1. Bring a large pot of water to a boil. Cook the pasta according to the package directions, stopping about 3 minutes short of the recommended cooking time so that it's al dente.

2. Drain and rinse the pasta and set it aside. Set a large sauté pan over medium heat. (I reuse my pasta pot since it's ceramic and can also go in the oven.)

3. Add the olive oil and onions and sauté with a pinch of salt, stirring occasionally, for about 6 minutes, until they're soft and translucent. Add the garlic and stir for another minute or two.

4. Add the broth, butternut squash cubes, tamari, mustard, paprika, salt, and pepper. Bring everything to a boil over high heat, then reduce to a simmer and cover. Cook for about 7 minutes, until the squash is tender when you poke it with a fork.

5. Preheat the oven to 350°F.

6. Remove the pot from the heat, take off the lid, and let the mixture sit so it gets cool enough to transfer to a blender.

7. While it's cooling, make the crumble topping. Simply place the almond meal, thyme, paprika, nutritional yeast, salt, and olive oil in a bowl and use a fork to mix them together. Set aside.

8. Place the sauce ingredients in a blender and add the almond milk, lemon juice, and nutritional yeast. Puree until silky smooth. Taste and add salt and pepper if you want.

9. Add the pasta to whatever dish you're gonna bake it in. A 2-quart baking dish (approx. 8 inch by 8 inch) would be just the thing. Note: It will seem soupy, but it will thicken up when it bakes so don't freak out.

10. Sprinkle the topping over the pasta.

11. Bake in the oven for about 30 minutes, until it's bubbly and golden brown.

12. Let this cool for a few minutes before serving. Leftovers of this are so superb, you might even call them the *bestovers*.

AFTER [PARTY] THOUGHT:

While, yes, this dish is creamy and orangey dreamy as it is, don't hesitate to green it up. My jam is to add 1 cup of frozen peas and 1 cup of frozen broccoli to the pot of boiling pasta at the very end of the pasta's cook time, plus 1 to 3 cups of fresh chopped kale, which I stir right into the pot with the sauce and pasta before baking.

WHEN YOU NEED TO COOK FOR YOUR FAMILY FULL OF PICKY EATERS

There's a reason Build-a-Bear stores at the mall are always jam-packed—because teddies are timeless. But also because DIYing helps kids feel empowered and allows mommies and daddies to catch their breath. Contrary to popular belief, the best way to cook for opinionated eaters is *not* to make a different meal for each family member but rather to put out build-your-own options for everyone to customize to their liking. So what follows are deconstructed meals everyone can DIY and will LUV.

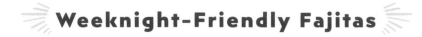

Weeknight-Friendly Fajitas

I used to get giddy every time my family would go to Chili's after seeing a movie because I got to "cook dinner," i.e., assemble stuff in tortillas and make a mess. My mom loved it because she didn't have to clean up the mess. My dad loved it because he loves napping in movie theaters. It was a victory all around. Just like these fajitas will be.

SERVES 4

FILLING

1 white onion, cut into thin slices

2 bell peppers (you pick the colors)

1 head of cauliflower

1 cup mushrooms

2 tablespoons olive or avocado oil

1 tablespoon chili powder (less if you don't like spice)

1 teaspoon cumin

½ teaspoon sweet paprika

¼ teaspoon garlic powder

¼ teaspoon onion powder

1 teaspoon sea salt or pink salt

GUAC-ISH

2 ripe avocados

Juice of 1 lime

½ teaspoon sea salt or pink salt

Fresh cilantro (optional)

CASHEW SOUR CREAM (OPTIONAL BUT DIVINE)

1 cup raw cashews, soaked in hot water for up to 2 hours

1 tablespoon freshly squeezed lemon juice

¼ teaspoon sea or pink salt

MAIN DISH

1 package of tortillas or a bunch of collard greens

1 15-ounce can of vegetarian refried beans, pinto beans, or black beans

1. Decide whether your family needs an additional protein or if beans are enough. If you're going to make an additional protein like Camo Tofu (page 48), TGIT (page 47), or meat, do what you need to do to start preparing that.

2. For your veggies, preheat the oven to 425°F. Line two baking sheets with parchment paper.

3. Wash the bell peppers and slice them. Wash the cauliflower and chop it into small florets. Clean the mushrooms and slice them. Add the veggies to a big bowl and toss them with the olive oil, chili powder, cumin, paprika, garlic powder, onion powder, and salt.

4. Spread the veggies on the baking sheets. Roast the veggies for about 20 minutes, popping in halfway to move them around so they cook evenly.

5. Make your Guac-ish (which I call because it's the easiest guac; I feel weird even calling it guacamole) by smashing the flesh from both avocados in a bowl with a fork. Add the lime juice, salt, and cilantro, if using (if your other half hates cilantro, like Jesse does, leave it on the side).

6. Optional step: Blend your cashew sour cream if you're making it. (Note that the cashews should be soaked in order to make this so you have to plan a little bit ahead.) Drain the cashews. Place them in a blender, along with ½ cup water, the lemon juice, and salt. Blend on your blender's highest speed until creamy.

7. If time allows, empty the can of beans into a small pan or pot set over medium heat. Stir until they start steaming and are at your desired temperature.

   To heat tortillas you have not one but three awesome options:

   a. Stove: Add tortillas, one by one, to a dry (no oil) skillet over medium heat and cook them for about 30 seconds on each side.

   b. Oven: Heat your oven to 350°F. Wrap a stack of five-ish tortillas in a packet of aluminum foil and cook for 15 to 20 minutes, until heated through.

   c. Microwave: Place five-ish tortillas on a micro-safe plate and cover them with a damp paper towel. Zap 'em in 30-second bursts until they are warm to the touch.

8. Your veggies should be done now, so remove them from the oven.

9. Optional step: Finish cooking the extra protein.

10. Lay everything out on the table for each person to DIY their meal.

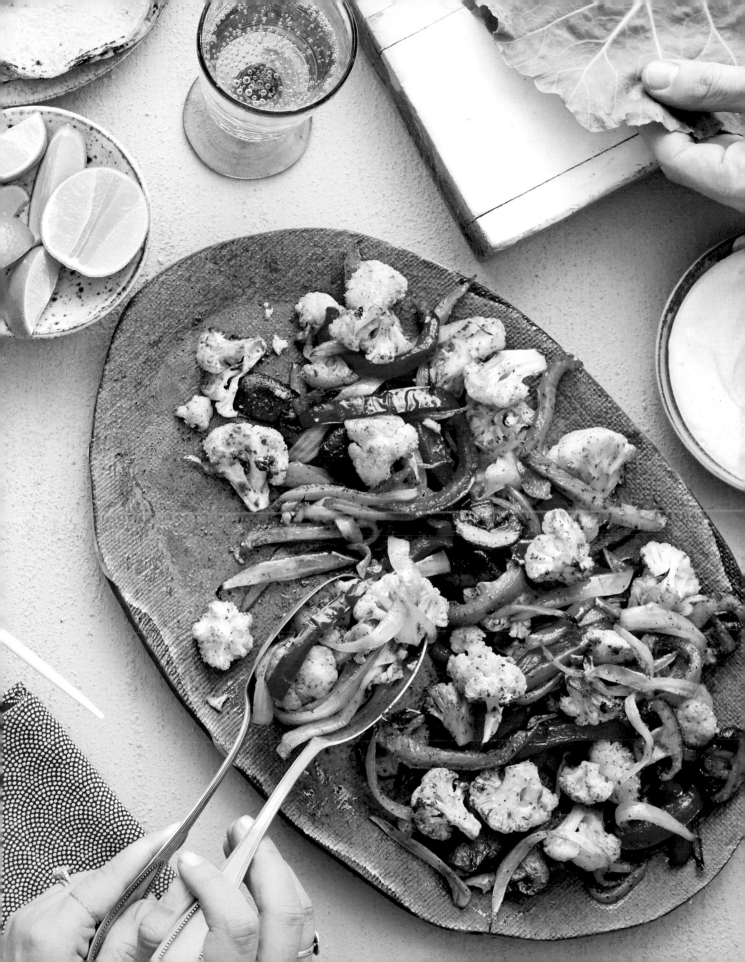

Customizable Chickpea Pizza

I believe that we all have the power to bring whatever we want into our life. Call it manifesting or call it picking your own toppings, and call this an inspirational blurb or a recipe intro, but this pizza is both a spiritual and a scrumptious experience that everyone can customize to achieve their wildest pizza-craving dreams without infringing on your pizza-craving dreams.

SERVES 2 (OR HALVE OR DOUBLE THIS)

CRUST

1½ cups chickpea flour

1 teaspoon sea salt or pink salt

¼ teaspoon onion powder (optional but yum)

¼ teaspoon garlic powder (optional but yum)

1 tablespoon extra-virgin olive oil

SUGGESTED (OPTIONAL) TOPPINGS

Tomato sauce (from a jar)

Dairy or nondairy cheese of your preference

Plants (see page 74)

1. Preheat the oven to 450°F.
2. In a medium or large bowl, mix together the flour, salt, onion powder (if using), garlic powder (if using), olive oil, and 1 cup water.
3. If you want to make two single-serving pizzas, take the smallest baking tray you have and line it with parchment paper. If you don't have a small baking tray, just use what you have, which might mean one double-serving pizza on your larger baking tray (also lined with parchment). No prob, everyone can still customize their half.
4. Spread the batter (which will be wet, not pliable like normal dough) out on your parchment paper and use a spatula to level it out so it's as even as you can make it.
5. Bake for 10 minutes.

NOTE: Read the tomato sauce jar label! Don't buy one that snuck sugar in there—you're sweet enough already.

HEALTHY EATING SUCKS.

"You killed it with this one! It was beyond what I had expected. The wet batter did worry me, but it ended up perfect. I made it for my friend and her fam who are skeptical about this kind of stuff, but they LOVED IT!" —JW

6. While it's baking, prepare your toppings. Open your tomato sauce if you're using it, chop and sauté any veggies you have lying around, or heat up a veggie burger.

7. If you're going to use a cheese, dairy or dairy-less, whip that out, too.

8. Once your pizza's baked for 10 minutes, remove it from the oven and top it with the tomato sauce, dairy or dairy-free cheese, veggies, or veggie burger, and put it back in the oven for 7 minutes.

9. Remove, cut, sprinkle with fresh basil if you have it, and enjoy.

I typically dig through my fridge and see what I can find. If my fridge is barren, I'll run to the nearest grocery store and grab an assortment of already-cut raw, grilled, or sautéed salad bar veggies.

My top pizza toppings are:

Spinach

Onion

Bell pepper

Garlic

Broccoli

Cauliflower

Mushrooms

BBQ Baked Tofu Cubes (page 49)

A veggie burger, cut up

Fresh basil (or pesto, such as Red Peppa Pesto on page 209 or Besto Pesto on page 200 or 212)

 LEFTOVERS ARE THE BESTOVERS:

Just like regular unhealthy pizza, this healthy pizza reheats well in an oven or tastes good, like the classic -za, cold out of the fridge.

WHEN YOU'RE COOKING FOR THAT CUTIE YOU SWIPED RIGHT FOR AND DON'T WANT TO BE TOO BLOATED TO DO STUFF AFTER DINNER

Cooking for a new crush can be a lot of pressure. My first time cooking for Jesse involved me peeling my finger instead of my zucchini and gushing blood as I woozily greeted him at the door. Your first time will be a heck of a lot different when you make your honey this Avocadodisiac Creamy Pasta, assuming you make sure the knife only cuts the avocado (which, by the way, has had an aphrodisiac reputation as far back as the Aztecs). Serve it with sexy sparkling and great-for-your-gut-and-lady-parts kombucha in a wineglass (or just wine . . . in a wineglass) and follow it with my "Sexy Can I Drizzle This Magic Chocolate Sauce" (page 79).

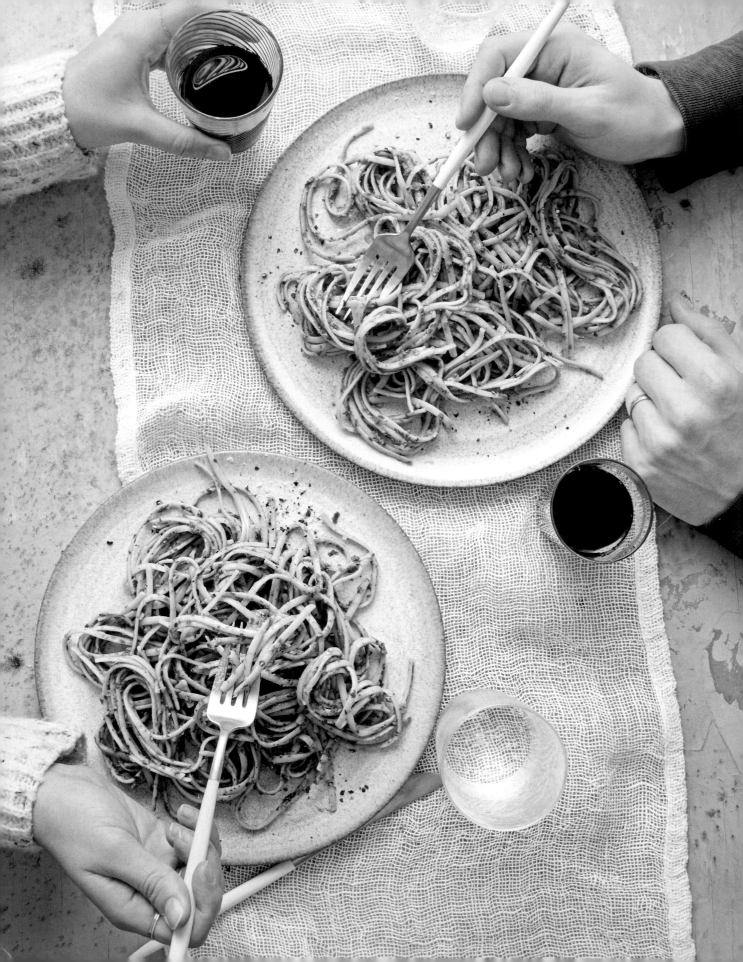

Avocadodisiac Creamy Pasta

You know those gals who prance around wearing minimal makeup with their hair in a seemingly effortless bun with just the cutest amount of messiness? I'm pretty sure their secret to natural but jaw-dropping beauty is "less is more," which is the exact secret to this effortless but jaw-dropping date-night dinner. It looks and tastes like you took a gap year studying pasta in Italy but comes together with a simple six ingredients thrown casually in a food processor.

SERVES 2

Protein of your choice (optional)

1 8-ounce package of your favorite pasta (enough for 2 to 3 servings)

1 cup fresh basil, tightly packed

1 cup raw spinach, tightly packed

1 ripe large avocado (or 2 small ones)

2 garlic cloves, raw or roasted

½ teaspoon salt, plus more for serving

Juice of ½ lemon

Freshly ground black pepper

1. Decide whether you're going to make a protein. If you are, start making that.
2. Boil water to cook the pasta according to the package's directions.
3. While the pasta's cooking, combine the basil, spinach, avocado, garlic, salt, lemon juice, and 1 tablespoon water in a food processor and blend until a creamy sauce is formed. You may need to add another tablespoon of water if the avocado isn't wildly creamy.
4. Mix the sauce with the cooked and drained pasta and then mix in or top with the optional protein.
5. For an extra flair, drizzle some good olive oil on top and sprinkle with freshly ground black pepper and an extra pinch of salt because you fancy!

HEALTHY EATING ~~SUCKS~~:

"My husband licked the bowl." **—KB**

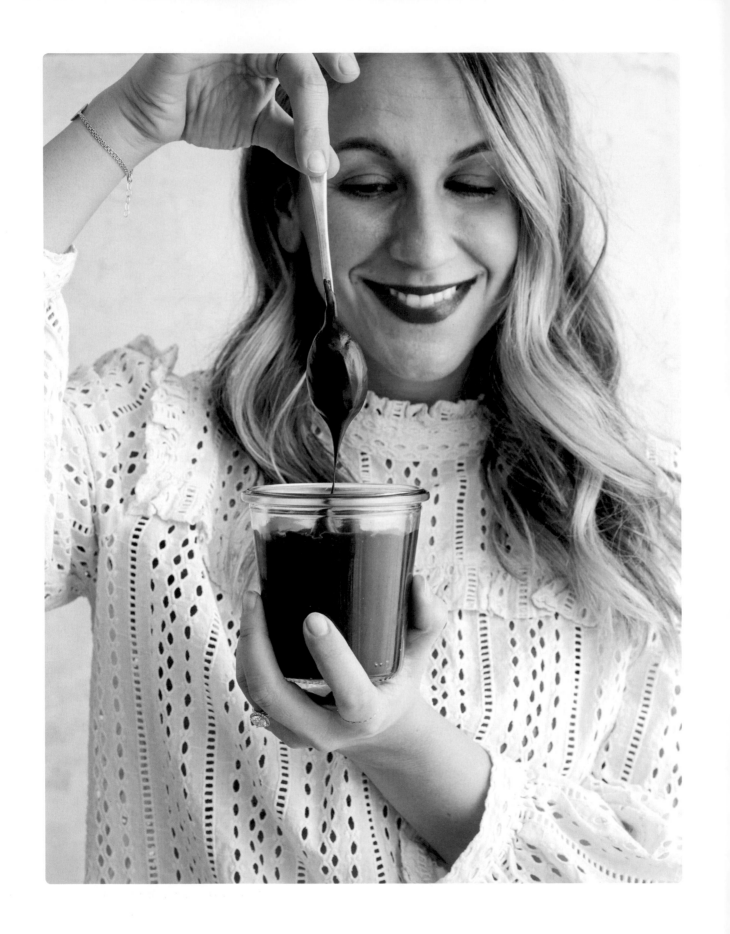

"Sexy Can I Drizzle This Magic Chocolate Sauce"

You know that bottle of chocolate sauce you have stashed away for chocolate emergencies like a culinary Neosporin? Ditch it like a dirty Band-Aid because this shizzle is the best to drizzle on any and most things.

MAKES ABOUT 1 CUP

¼ cup coconut oil, refined (so your sauce doesn't taste like a piña colada)

½ cup cacao powder or cocoa powder (see page 315)

¼ cup maple syrup

1 teaspoon vanilla extract

Pinch of sea salt

1. In a small saucepan over low heat, melt the coconut oil. Use a wooden spoon or spatula to encourage it to melt over the heat.
2. Once it has melted, turn off the heat and add the cacao powder, maple syrup, vanilla, and salt. Stir to combine really well. Watch it turn into an awesome chocolate sauce.
3. Pour it into a glass jar to drizzle on popcorn, bowls of fruit, banana ice cream, oatmeal, apple nachos, fingers, pancakes, etc.
4. It should stay fresh on your counter for 7 to 10 days.

AFTER [PARTY] THOUGHT:

If your sauce thickens up too much, use a double-boiler method to bring it back to drizzle status. Double boiling means filling a small pot with water and placing it on the stove, bringing the water to a simmer, and then placing a metal bowl on top of the pot. Using a spatula, mix your chocolate to remelt it.

Zzzz

WHEN YOU WAKE UP IN THE FANTASY SUITE, OR OTHERWISE EXECUTE A SEXY BREAKFAST IN BED

I don't know what goes down for breakfast when the *Bachelor* contestants wake up in the fantasy suite, but I like to imagine them eating these sexy B-in-B dishes that won't give you unsexy heartburn.

Lemon Chia–Not–Poppy Seed Mini Muffins

What does it say about my youth that the mini lemon poppy seed muffins my mom brought home from Big Y each Monday was a high point? Ah, screw psychoanalysis and let's celebrate that I've re-created a peak childhood moment in a way that pleases current Talia's body. These natural lemon cuties made with chia seeds have the same stick-in-your-teeth effect as those past-life muffins, except they also pack in omega-3 fats, fiber, antioxidants, iron, and calcium, without butter, crappy sugar, or glutenous white flour to rain on the muffin parade.

MAKES 24 MINI MUFFINS OR ABOUT 10 LARGE MUFFINS

FOR THE CHIA GEL

¼ cup chia seeds

DRY INGREDIENTS

2 cups almond flour

¼ teaspoon sea salt

½ teaspoon baking soda

1 tablespoon cardamom (optional)

WET INGREDIENTS

⅓ cup maple syrup

1 teaspoon vanilla extract

2 tablespoons lemon zest (from about 2 lemons)

2 tablespoons freshly squeezed lemon juice (from ½ to 1 whole lemon)

1 tablespoon coconut oil, melted

1. Preheat the oven to 350°F. Spritz a muffin tin tray with coconut oil or line it with muffin cups.

2. Make the chia gel by adding ½ cup water and 3 tablespoons chia seeds to a large measuring cup or a bowl. Use a fork to stir well so the seeds spread out in the cup. Set aside.

3. In a large bowl, combine the almond meal, salt, baking soda, and cardamom, if using, and mix well. If your almond meal has some clumps in it, break them up.

4. Say hi to your chia gel. Use a fork to mix it again so all the seeds become gelled (you'll see what I mean). Set aside.

5. In a small bowl, mix together the maple syrup, vanilla, lemon zest, lemon juice, and melted coconut oil.

6. Transfer the wet ingredients to the bowl with the dry ones and stir in the chia gel.

7. Mix well so no dry flour is left behind.

8. Add the remaining 1 tablespoon chia seeds into the batter to give these muffins that "poppy seed" effect.

9. Fill each muffin cup about two-thirds of the way with batter. Note: They won't dome like typical muffins so what you see before they go in the oven is what you'll also see when they come out.

10. Bake for 20 to 25 minutes. They're done when the tops are just lightly golden.

11. Remove from the oven and let cool for at least 5 minutes—they'll harden up a bit!

12. Store leftovers covered in the fridge.

HEALTHY EATING SUCKS:

"My hubs liked the chia crunch—and he's
anti–poppy seeds!"—**MD**

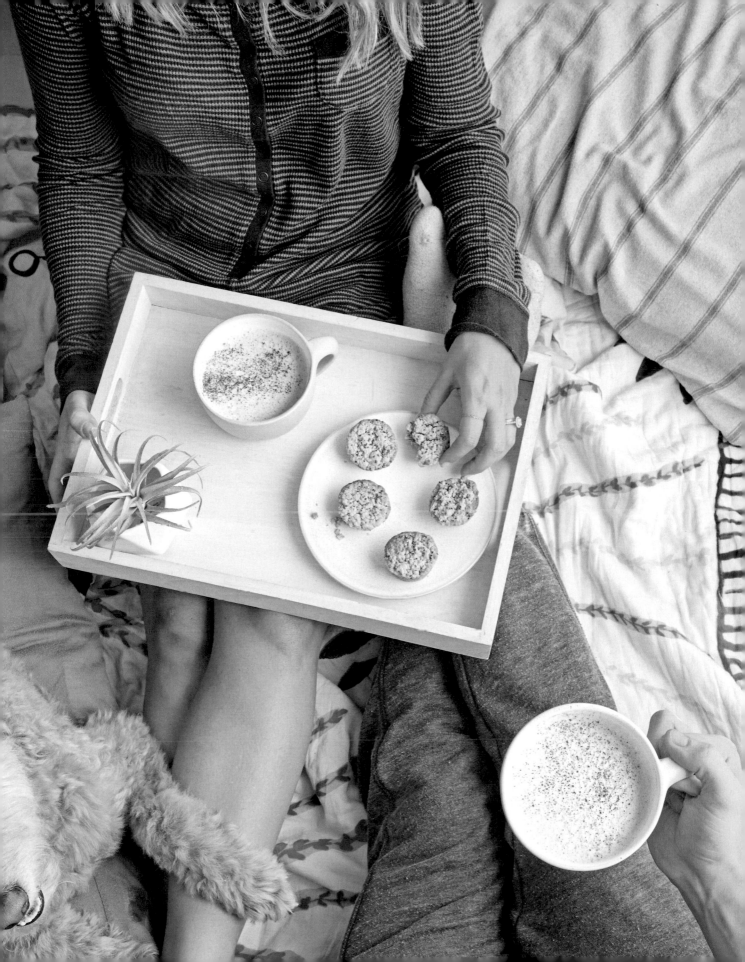

Jesse's Secret Creamy, Dreamy Pumpkin Oatmeal

Many years ago, during that serious-but-not-yet-living-together-but-toothbrushes-at-one-another's-apartments period of our relationship, Jesse learned to cook. His studio apartment was situated directly on top of a huge Whole Foods, so our almost daily routine involved us meeting there after work, grabbing some plants, waiting in line for fifty minutes, and going upstairs to cook 'em. His first skill set was roasted veggies. After mastering the toss in olive oil plus salt (and random other swings and misses #cinnamonroastedonionsarenotgood), he conquered the stovetop with oatmeal for two. One winter morning he presented me with a decadent pumpkin oatmeal and I knew he was a keeper. As was his recipe. Where now the addition of cinnamon is more than welcomed.

SERVES 2

¾ cup almond milk

1 cup rolled oats

¾ cup pumpkin puree

1 tablespoon almond butter

1 teaspoon pumpkin pie spice

1 teaspoon vanilla extract

½ teaspoon cinnamon

2 tablespoons maple syrup

1. In a small saucepan, add the almond milk and ¾ cup water. Increase the heat and bring the liquid to a boil.

2. Add the rolled oats. Return to a boil and simmer for about 5 minutes, until the liquid's mostly gone, stirring along the way.

3. Mix in the pumpkin puree and reduce the heat to low.

4. Add the almond butter, pumpkin pie spice, vanilla, cinnamon, and maple syrup. Mix well.

5. Raise the heat to medium and simmer for another 5 to 10 minutes, stopping before it's 100 percent dry—Jesse's secret to keeping it creamy and dreamy.

6. Serve warm and with love. Consider topping this with Very Present-able Roasted Pecans (page 260).

AFTER [PARTY] THOUGHT:

This oatmeal can be made ahead of time, and can easily scale to any size group. It reheats favorably, too, making it a "when you make any, make many" kind of meal that you can later bring back to coziness in the microwave or on the stove with a splash of almond milk.

Oatmeal master Jesse wants you to know that this recipe also works with 1 cup of frozen berries added in place of canned pumpkin, cutting the pumpkin pie spice.

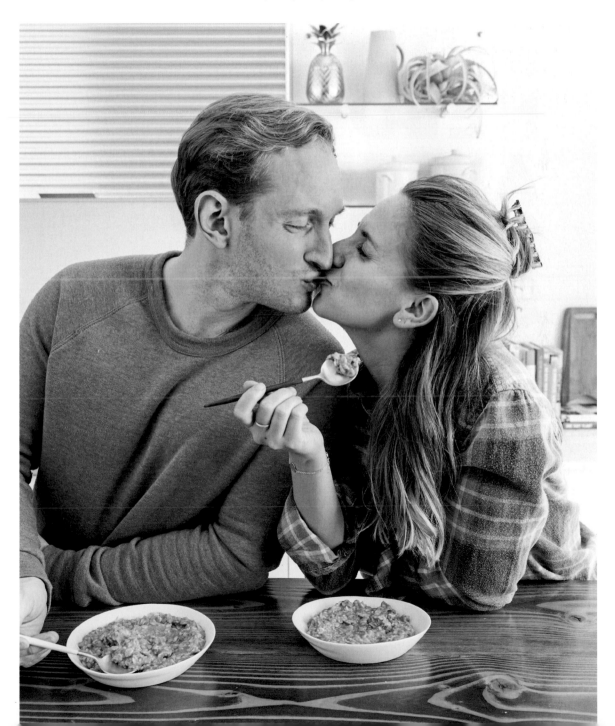

WHEN YOUR KIDDOS NEED AN AFTER-SCHOOL SNACK

It's good to grow out of little kid things like sucking thumbs or peeing in beds, but I'm a firm believer in Peter-Panning after-school snacks (never growing out of them, that is). However, adulthood means saying goodbye to crap-filled goldfish my sister would dive face and fist first into and sleeves of processed graham crackers with corn-syrup-whipped peanut butter I'd eat until I had no more room for dinner. Here are two snacks that prove age is just a number and healthy food is just as good as crappy food.

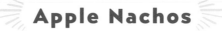

Apple Nachos

Apple nachos are a splendid edible project for kids trying to get more food on their hands, as well as a photogenic snack for adults trying to get more nutrients into their lives. (And more likes on social media.) They're also healthy, delicious, endlessly customizable, and a true party with plants.

SERVES 2 BUT EASY TO DOUBLE, TRIPLE, OR HALVE

2 washed apples, whatever variety your eaters like/your market has

¼ to ½ cup gooey topping(s), like Caramel Fit for a Date (page 188), "Sexy Can I Drizzle This Magic Chocolate Sauce" (page 79), tahini melted in the microwave, or room-temperature peanut butter or almond butter

1 to 2 handfuls of chunky toppings— raisins, goji berries, chocolate chips, carob chips, granola, coconut flakes

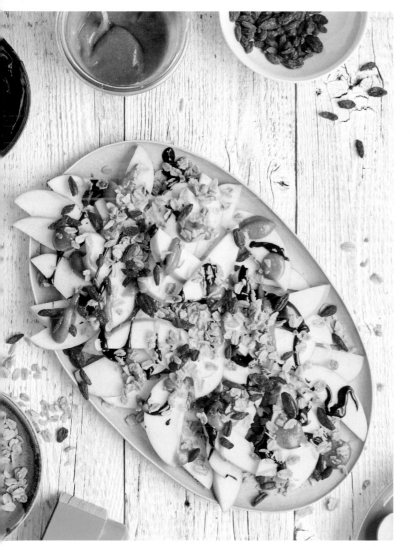

1. Slice the apples thinly and spread them out on a large plate or serving platter.
2. Use a fork to drizzle gooey topping(s) on top.
3. Use your hands to add the chunky topping(s).
4. Yum!

Cheeseisn'ts

I originally titled these "Cheesenots," but during my cookbook shoot it dawned on me that "not" isn't quite the opposite of "it." So I hollered out to my photo team, "Hey, guys, what's the opposite of 'its'?!" and Drew, while executing *Chopped*-level onion chopping skills for my chili (You'll TouchDOWN This Pumpkin Black Bean Chili, page 249—yum!), shouted back, "Isn't?" and this recipe's name was finalized. Cheeseisn'ts honor their orange inspiration, except these get their hue from nutrition-packed (and mega-cheap) canned pumpkin and vitamin B–loaded nutritional yeast. They work as a plate-to-mouth snack, or you can take a plate–to–peanut butter (organic and with no added oil or sugar)–to mouth detour.

SERVES 2 TO 3 AS A SNACK

½ cup canned pumpkin puree

¾ cup oat flour

½ teaspoon sea salt or pink salt

2 tablespoons nutritional yeast

¼ teaspoon garlic powder

Pinch of cayenne or chipotle powder for spice (optional)

1. Preheat the oven to 350°F. Line a baking sheet with parchment paper.
2. In a large bowl, combine the pumpkin puree, oat flour, salt, nutritional yeast, garlic powder, and cayenne if using. Stir well and form into a dough.
3. Transfer the dough to the prepared baking sheet.
4. Top the dough with another sheet of parchment paper.
5. Use a rolling pin to roll the dough into a thin, uniform layer.
6. *Gently* peel off the top parchment paper and use a pizza cutter or a knife to cut the dough into bite-size squares. I use a chopstick to poke a hole in the middle of each cracker for the full Cheese-It effect. This is optional but fun.
7. Bake for 15 minutes, then flip the crackers with a spatula to bake them evenly. If you didn't cut them all the way through the first time around, you might need to break them up now.
8. Put them back in the oven for about 10 minutes, until they're dry and crispy.
9. Let the crackers cool and harden up, then dive in.
10. Store leftovers in a sealed container at room temperature for up to 5 days.

AFTER [PARTY] THOUGHT:

Other awesome after-school/work snacks are Bananagrams (page 258), Fooled Ya Black Bean Brownies (page 279), Go Blondies (page 243), Nice Crispy Treats (page 197), Chia Pudding (page 283), and any of the balls found on pages 255, 275, and 303.

WHEN Y'ALL ARE CRAVING THAI

Thai cravings happen. For me, they're all the Thai'm. For you, they might be someThai'ms. Here's my plant-packed pad Thai, which also makes lovely leftovers for another Thai'm.

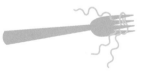

Pad Thai in No Thai'm

SERVES 2 TO 3

Camo Tofu (page 48)

SAUCE

Juice of 1 lime

2 tablespoons regular peanut butter

2 tablespoons tamari

1 tablespoon toasted sesame oil

1 teaspoon Sriracha, plus more to garnish

1½ teaspoons coconut sugar

½ teaspoon ginger powder

2 garlic cloves, peeled and chopped

DISH

1 14-ounce package of pad Thai noodles or Asian rice noodles

1 cup edamame (fresh or frozen)

1 or 2 medium sweet potatoes (peeled if not organic), spiralized

1 or 2 zucchini, spiralized

1½ teaspoons coconut or avocado oil

1 cup shredded/cut-up red cabbage

1 bell pepper (any color), cut into small slices or chunks

Cilantro (optional)

1. Make the Camo Tofu.
2. In a small bowl, blend the lime juice, peanut butter, tamari, sesame oil, Sriracha, coconut sugar, ginger, and garlic and set aside.
3. Bring a pot of water to a boil and cook the pad Thai noodles according to the package's instructions. Drain, rinse, and set aside.
4. If you're using frozen edamame, boil, drain, and set aside.
5. Put the sweet potato and zucchini noodles in a sauté pan over medium heat. Add the coconut oil, stirring frequently so the noodles cook evenly.
6. When the noodles start to get soft, add the cabbage, bell peppers, and boiled and drained edamame to the pan and cook until the veggies are your desired texture.
7. In a large bowl, place the sautéed veggies, pad Thai noodles, sauce, and Camo Tofu and mix. Add cilantro if your family likes it.
8. Serve, garnished with extra Sriracha and cilantro, if using.

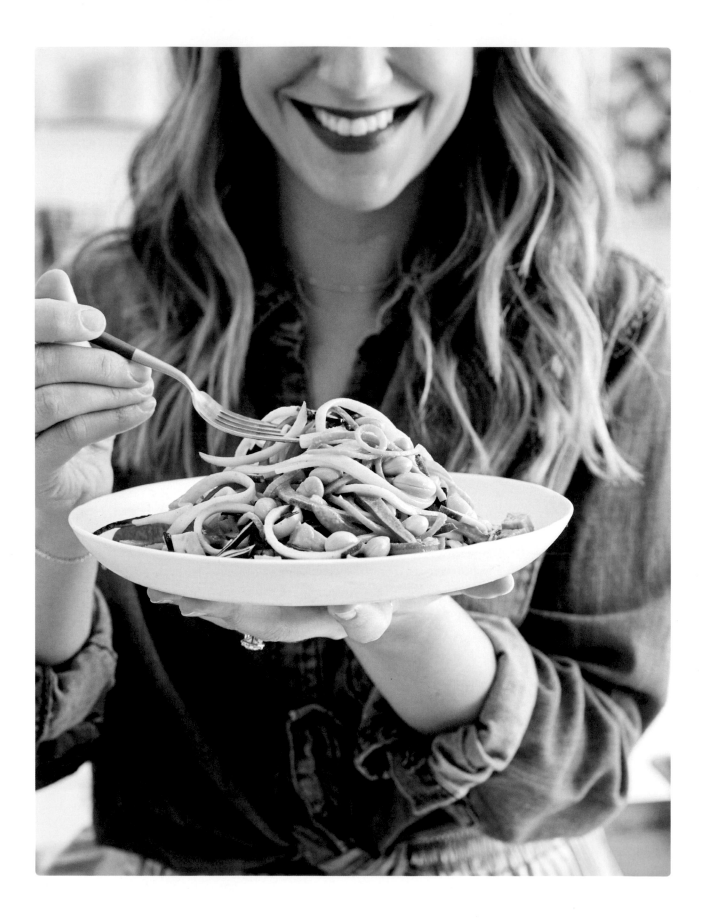

WHEN YOU WANT TO UPGRADE DELIVERY

By no means am I justifying daily delivery, but I am saying there *is* a way to healthify those "just bring me some damn food" evenings. Here's how to hack the system:

Step 1—Order with an emphasis on veggies and protein. Ask for many veggies, extra veggies, all the veggies, go crazy. (No eye contact when ordering means no judgment.)

Ordering Thai, Indian, or Chinese food? "Light on the oil, please" or ask for sauces on the side. Ordering Japanese? Get veggie sushi with brown rice, or maki rolls, which have less rice, alongside edamame—an A+ plant protein. Top pizza with every vegetable they've got and don't be shy about nixing the cheese. For Mexican, it's the bestican to go for veggie fajitas or tacos (with soft corn tortillas instead of flour). Tack on a side of vegetarian beans for extra fun to toot! I mean boot.

Step 2—Get cracking on your upgrade! Sweet Potato Wedgies (page 97) pair perfectly with a vegburger and Really Nice Cauliflower Rice (page 94) or Hit Me with Your Best Sauce Quinoa (page 96) complement cuisines that prominently feature rice. Supplement that blah romaine salad with chopped kale or spinach and, if pizza's on its way, chop up and lightly sauté every stray veggie you can find.

Step 3—Delivery arrives; give a nice tip. (A really nice one. Speaking from my experience as a college pizza delivery girl, it means the difference between riding back to pizza HQ blasting Britney Spears or Evanescence.)

Step 4.1—Top pizza with your veggie medley and/or favorite cheese and pop it in the oven for a few minutes at 400°F to bring the temperature back up.

Step 4.2—Take a slotted spoon and scoop the delivery onto your rice or quinoa, allowing any excess sauce to strain out.

Step 4.3—Replace the taco or fajita toppings with your sexier ones. Douse with high-quality hot sauce.

Really Nice Cauliflower Rice
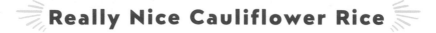

Cauliflower rice is the actual coolest thing since sliced bread. It's cool not only because it makes you feel like you hacked the starch-side system but because it allows you to get a hit of nutrition without even trying.

MAKES 4 SERVINGS

1 head of cauliflower

1 tablespoon olive oil or to taste

Salt and freshly ground black pepper
to taste

Other spices, fresh herbs, tamari, and
nutritional yeast/pecorino to taste

1. Chop the cauliflower so it easily packs into your food processor. (Perfection is hardly necessary here.) Wash it and let excess water drain out of the colander.

2. Place the cauliflower chunks in a food processor and pulse until they've broken down into a texture that resembles rice. Pause the food processor intermittently to scrape down the sides.

3. Heat the olive oil in a skillet over medium heat.

4. Add the cauliflower rice, salt, pepper, and any other seasonings you're using. Use a lid to cover the rice so the cauliflower steams and becomes more tender. Cook for about 5 minutes.

AFTER [PARTY] THOUGHT:

Want the second coolest thing since sliced bread? Or the thing
that's tied with the coolest thing since sliced bread? Make sweet
potato rice! Follow the same instructions as above to process
2 sweet potatoes into the texture of rice. Sauté this magic in
a pan with 1 tablespoon of olive or coconut oil plus salt and
pepper to taste for about 7 minutes, and then shout SWEET!

Left to right: Really Nice Cauliflower
Rice, Hit Me with Your Best Sauce
Quinoa, Sweet Potato Wedgies

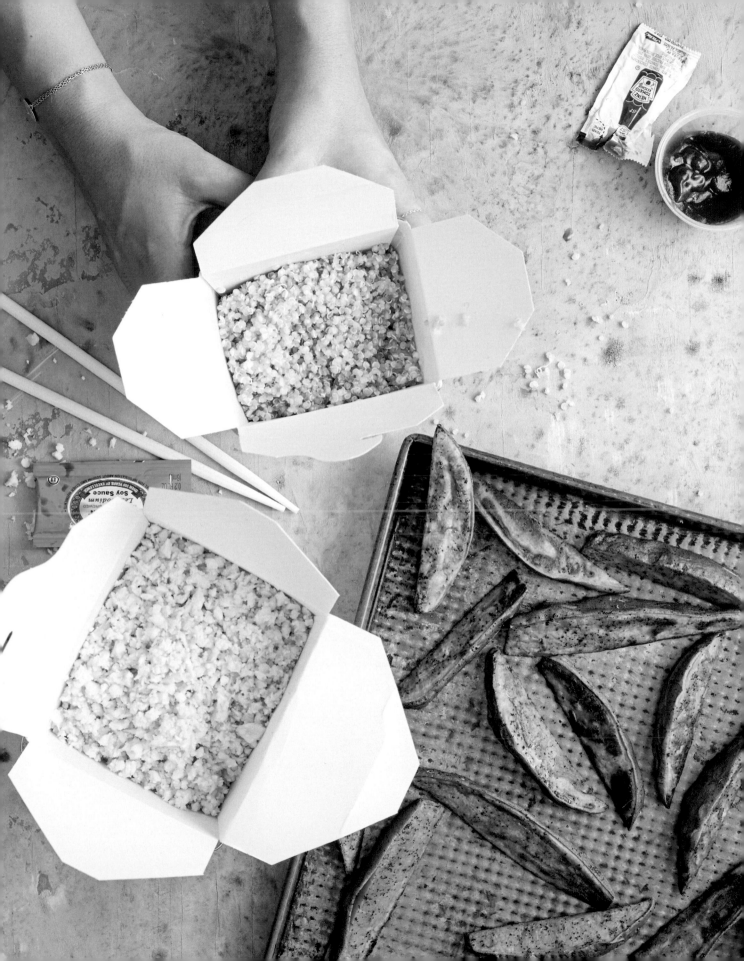

Hit Me with Your Best Sauce Quinoa

Plain, fluffy quinoa is like a nineteen-year-old aspiring actress moving from small-town Kentucky to Hollywood—a bundle of hope and willingness to be molded into the superstar she's meant to be. In my home, quinoa plays the part of the quirky gluten-free and protein-rich best friend to fajitas, salads, delivery curry, and random leftovers.

SERVES 4 (EASY TO DOUBLE OR HALVE)

1 cup quinoa, any color

2 cups water

1. If you have a fine-mesh strainer, use it to rinse the quinoa. If you don't have a fine-mesh strainer, don't sweat it and just place your quinoa in a medium pot on the stove.
2. Add the water to the pot and bring to a boil over high heat.
3. Once the water is boiling, give the quinoa a stir and reduce the heat to low so it lightly simmers, uncovered, for about 15 minutes.
4. Turn off the heat and give the quinoa another stir to fluff it like a pillow.

Sweet Potato Wedgies

When I met Jesse, I learned that he has three nonnegotiables: a night's sleep must never be shorter than eight and a half hours, red lipstick shouldn't exist, and anything called fries must be crispy. Number one he takes care of, number two I ignore because no man can come between me and a bold lip, and number three I've worked diligently on. The problem with making healthy sweet potato fries that are as crispy as unhealthy sweet potato fries is that it's, well, not possible (without extreme soaking methods, exotic coating ingredients, and way too much attention to detail). Solution: I stopped calling them "fries" and started calling them what they are—sweet potato wedgies.

SERVES 2 (ASSUMING 1 POTATO PER PERSON)

2 large sweet potatoes

1 tablespoon extra-virgin olive oil

½ teaspoon sea salt

½ teaspoon chili powder (optional; more or less depending on how spicy you like it)

1. Preheat the oven to 425°F.
2. Wash the sweet potatoes and cut off the tips of both ends.
3. Position the sweet potatoes horizontally on a cutting board and cut them in half.
4. Cut each half in half again, then put each on its side and cut it into wedges. Place them in a large bowl.
5. When you've cut all of your wedgies, add the olive oil, salt, and the chili powder, if using, and toss all around to coat evenly.
6. Spread the wedgies on a rimmed baking sheet (no need for parchment paper this time) and roast for 20 minutes. Pop into the oven, move the wedgies around with a spatula or wooden spoon to help them cook evenly, and cook for another 10 minutes.
7. Remove from the oven and turn on the oven broiler. When it's heated up, slide the sweet potato pan back in and broil on the top rack for 4 to 5 minutes, keeping a close eye (and nose) on them so they're just charred but not burned.
8. Serve warm.
9. Store leftovers in the fridge.

HEALTHY EATING WHEN YOU'RE HOME ALONE
How to Not Eat Everything But the Kitchen Sink When You Work from Home (or Just Live There)

Sometimes when I'm dicing an onion I look at my knife and think, "I'm casually holding a potential murder weapon." Then I realize that maybe I watch a little too much true crime. But *then* I conclude that it's *my* decision to make the knife a partner in a healthy dinner versus a *Dexter*-esque partner in crime, and that's empowering.

The same thing can be said about a fridge and pantry full of food sitting in our homes at all time. Only you can choose to make that food a "danger zone" or just a place to keep it fresh and organized. Since I work from home, I could eat out of my fridge and pantry all day long. Nobody would know. My only co-worker wouldn't judge me—though he might eat any food I drop right off the ground. (He's a dog.)

Here are two ways I refrain from turning my home into a 24/7 Vegas-style buffet:

I eat regular meals. Just like a normal person working in an office takes a lunch break some hours after breakfast and then heads out for dinner, and does not saunter over to the communal fridge every five minutes, braless and in sweatpants, to grab another bite, I hold myself to the same standards. (Except for the bra because why would I do that to myself?)

I worship ramekins: I first got my hands on these small ceramic bowls in culinary school, where they held our mises.[7] They are palm-size, which happens to be a perfect snack size. I use ramekins to portion out cut-up fruit, nuts, granola, popcorn, crackers, chia pudding.

I love what I do: What? Career advice in a plant food book? Stay in your lane, Talia. Well, considering that finding fulfillment from my day-to-day doings distracts me from needing to fill an empty void with fridge food, I feel like that's eating advice I'm qualified to pass along.

How to Make Cooking Time < Eating Time When You're Eating Stag

I have a rule that when I'm eating dinner alone, cooking time cannot surpass eating time. Two reasons: It incentivizes me to s-l-o-w d-o-w-n as I eat because I don't want eating time to be less than prep time. It also permits me to do what I refer to as "bowlin'" and to utilize the crap out of my leftovers.

---

7 The pre-chopped or pre-portioned ingredients that maximize your efficiency. In case you want to learn some trivia: "Mise en place" is a French phrase that roughly translates to "everything in its place."

On "bowlin'":

When I enrolled in culinary school I was determined to learn how to kick ass in my kitchen. And I did. I learned (and ate) a lot, and came out of it thinking I was going to be a gourmet at-home chef. I imagined myself whipping up perfectly pureed and delicately garnished soups for my significant other's sick day, baking and frosting photogenic three-tiered cakes for family birthdays, and tossing salads that rival those at the Four Seasons. So when I found myself eating bowls of quinoa with pesto and some stray veggies for dinner, I was confused. Ditto when I noticed that I was drinking easy smoothies each morning.

But then I realized that gourmet doesn't always mean yay and simple food puts me in a better mood. I was intuitively doing something pretty cool: bowlin'. Bowlin' is perfect for when you don't want to fuss with three-dish meals, you don't want to deal with cleanup, and honestly, you just want to shove something tasty into your mouth. It's a super-duper easy way to eat filling meals without being a whiz in the kitchen (or a millionaire at the supermarket).

All you do is throw three or four ingredients in a bowl, and you've got a filling, nutritious, and tasty bowl o' goodness. My fail-proof formula is:

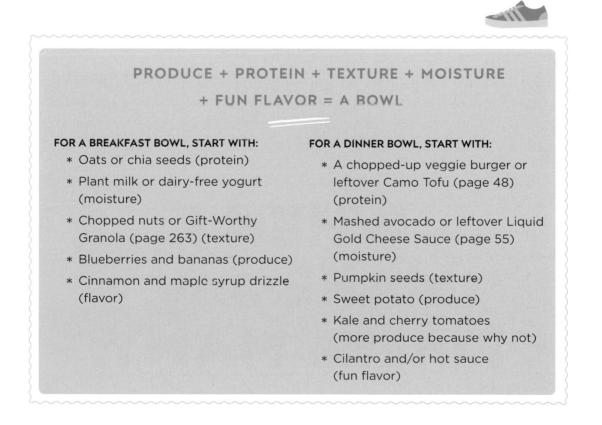

PRODUCE + PROTEIN + TEXTURE + MOISTURE + FUN FLAVOR = A BOWL

FOR A BREAKFAST BOWL, START WITH:

* Oats or chia seeds (protein)
* Plant milk or dairy-free yogurt (moisture)
* Chopped nuts or Gift-Worthy Granola (page 263) (texture)
* Blueberries and bananas (produce)
* Cinnamon and maple syrup drizzle (flavor)

FOR A DINNER BOWL, START WITH:

* A chopped-up veggie burger or leftover Camo Tofu (page 48) (protein)
* Mashed avocado or leftover Liquid Gold Cheese Sauce (page 55) (moisture)
* Pumpkin seeds (texture)
* Sweet potato (produce)
* Kale and cherry tomatoes (more produce because why not)
* Cilantro and/or hot sauce (fun flavor)

Sure, sometimes it's fun to make a restaurant-quality dinner. You plan it out, pull recipes from cookbooks, make a grocery list, throw on comfy clothes, hit up the store, blast bouncy tunes, and rock out as you cook something special. But most of the time, I prefer the time I take to cook to be less than the time I take to eat. You too? Perf. Then bowlin' is for you.

· ·

Food Porn Should Be X-Rated

Just like watching porn will not get you laid, drooling over food porn will not get you any healthier. If you're not familiar with food porn, it's when someone pampers, makes up, poses, shoots, and Photoshops their meal in the same way someone styles, pampers, makes up, posts, shoots, and Photoshops Kim Kardashian. That food ain't even *edible* a lot of the time. And being able to edit a sexy photo doesn't make anyone an expert on the inner workings of your unique body, no matter how seductive those bliss balls look.

· ·

On Making Leftovers the Bestovers

I am so anti-batch cooking you could call me the No Batch Bitch. The idea of spending my whole Sunday cooking when I could be, um, living seems as absurd as getting my fingernails painted in a color other than top coat when I know they'll just chip on my walk home from the salon. Instead, I implement this simple philosophy:

WHEN I MAKE any, I make MANY.

I double, triple, even quadruple every single thing that I make. Why get my booty into the kitchen, my hands covered in garlic, my kitchen coated in lemon juice, and my floor sprinkled with kale shavings just to create a onetime thing? When you make something, make many portions. If a recipe only calls for 1 cup of quinoa, cook 3. Portion out a third, use it in the recipe, and then save the leftover two-thirds. Sauce? Double it! Baked goods? Double them! (And freeze the leftovers.) The only thing that's not leftover-able is a smoothie. Everything else is fair game.

Leftovers can be the difference between eating crap and eating healthy. They can be the difference between eating when you're hungry or not eating when you're hungry (read: they're hanger-helpers).

Leftovers work in two ways. One, you can make and store dishes, like soups, salads, or pastas, that you can just heat up (or eat cold). Two, you can make and store leftover ingredients, like plain quinoa, roasted tempeh, or baked sweet potatoes, to use with other ingredients and make epic impromptu dishes on the fly.

Save everything.

Against Jesse's instincts or minimalist wishes, I will save anything edible. I don't care if that's 3 tablespoons of peas, 1/4 cup of quinoa, half a jar packed with pumpkin puree, or a small bite of a snack ball. (True story.) I always find myself using the stuff I save (in things like bowlin' dinners) and in turn, doing stuff I enjoy (things like bowling in alleys) in the extra time I saved.

Don't forget the lubrication.

In this book you'll find some dressings, spreads, and sauces. Commit those recipes to memory or at least commit to making many when you make any

so you always have some of them standing by in jars in your fridge to elevate your leftovers and your bowlin'. If you find yourself lube-less, though, don't panic. A drizzle of olive oil, lemon juice, tamari, or tahini can also elevate a leftover meal, maybe not into bestovers, but into greatovers.

Test-drive many vehicles.

Though forks and spoons are technically all you need to help leftovers travel to your mouth, I suggest you test out other vehicles as well. Leftover veggies and proteins go nicely over kale that you massaged with lemon juice plus a drizzle of olive oil and a couple of pinches of salt. Leftovers on top of quinoa is a true resurrection. Pizza crust (like the one in Customizable Chickpea Pizza, page 72), baked sweet potato, pasta, and quesadillas rock with tofu, tempeh, and random scraps of veggies. And when in doubt, or whenever you really want, just wrap 'em up—in a wrap.

Get your freezer in on the fun.

Your freezer can really take the plant party to the next level and help you eat healthfully next time you're too tired to cook dinner. Soups, chilis, and some casseroles freeze beautifully, as do extra grains, sauces, and legumes. If you have the space in your home and your budget, you could even get an extra freezer specifically for leftovers (I say wistfully from my 700-square-foot Brooklyn apartment).

Use glass to save your ass.

Tinted windows are cool if you're avoiding paparazzi—or the cops—but for leftovers? They're about as un-cool as it gets. As brain-boosting as your healthy diet might help you be, you're never going to remember what the heck is sitting in that old yogurt container, so store leftovers in glass. It's better for your food, the environment, and your wallet if you rinse out pasta sauce jars, pickle jars, and nut butter jars.

Divide and conquer.

As best as you can, portioning out your leftovers in individual containers can be a lifesaver. I'm not saying separate each layer of leftover lasagna into its own Tupperware, but if you have extra sweet potato, save it separately from the black beans. Also, only dress what you're going to wear—I mean eat! Don't put sauces on things you plan to save, as that will make those things not as tasty when you go back for them later.

WHEN YOU'RE EATING SOLO

What happens when you eat dinner alone stays in your belly after you eat dinner alone. And while that might be cereal, it could also be a High-Def TV Dinner (page 105), reminiscent of those trays of crappy plate dinners we see in old movies being eaten in front of even older TVs, but stuffed with every nutritious plant scrap I can find. This single meal can easily be doubled if a neighbor swings by or if you want to pre-make lunch tomorrow.

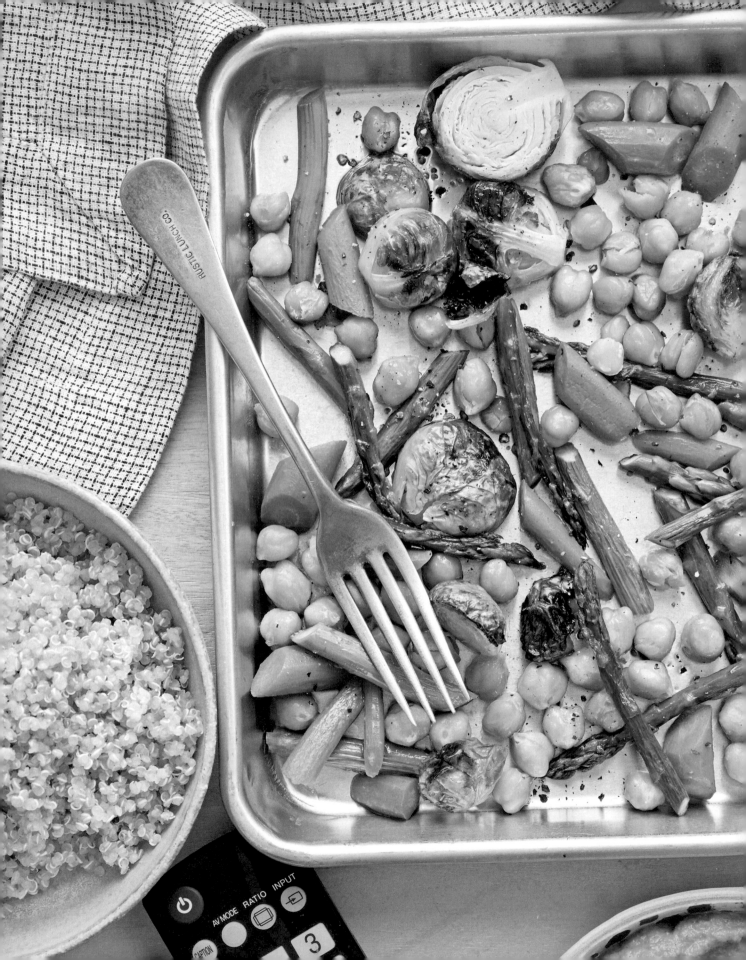

High-Def TV Dinner

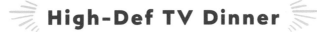

SERVES 2 TO 3 (OR 1 WITH SWEET LEFTOVERS!)

A PLANT PROTEIN, LIKE:

1 can chickpeas, black beans, white beans, kidney beans, or navy beans

1 package tofu, pressed and cubed

1 package tempeh, cubed

4 TO 8 CUPS VEGGIE MEDLEY, LIKE:

Onion, chopped

Garlic cloves, chopped

Sweet potato, washed and cubed

Squash (butternut, acorn), cubed

Brussels sprouts, washed and halved

Broccoli, washed and chopped

Cauliflower, washed and chopped

Fennel, washed and chopped

Carrots, washed, peeled, and chopped

Asparagus, washed and coarsely chopped (or kept whole)

Green beans, washed

Kale, washed and coarsely ripped off the stems (optional)

A SPICE, LIKE:

1 tablespoon chili powder, garlic powder, or curry powder

1 to 3 tablespoons olive oil or avocado oil

½ to 1 teaspoon sea salt or pink salt

Freshly ground black pepper to taste

Other spices (optional)

A SAUCE, LIKE:

Red Peppa Pesto (page 209)

Besto Pesto (page 212)

Tahini Miso Magic Sauce (page 273)

Liquid Gold Cheese Sauce (page 55)

A "VEHICLE," LIKE:

1 spread-eagle sweet potato

Steamed quinoa

Cooked plant-based pasta (optional)

1. Preheat the oven to 400°F.
2. Prepare your protein. If using tofu, press it. If using beans, drain and rinse and dry them. If using tempeh, chop it. Set aside.
3. In a large mixing bowl, add all the veggies (except the optional kale). Toss and add your protein. Sprinkle with chili powder, olive oil, salt, pepper, and any other spice you'd like. Toss well so everything gets coated.

4. Transfer the mixture onto one or two ungreased rimmed baking sheets (just depends on how many veggies you're using). Bake for 20 to 30 minutes. Don't hesitate to get in there and use a spatula to move the veggies around so they cook evenly. When there's about 10 minutes left, toss the kale, if using, with a splash of olive oil and sea salt. Add to a baking sheet.

5. Make a "vehicle"—a baked sweet potato, steamed quinoa, or pasta.

6. Make a sauce.

7. When your veggies are done, remove them from the oven.

8. Combine all of the components in a large bowl, a plate, or heck, even right on the baking sheet, and eat.

WHEN YOU NEED DESSERT FOR 1

No longer do stag desserts mean sad desserts. This single-portion Banana Ice Cream is about as much fun as one can have alone while keeping your clothes on. And this single cookie? Good enough to wish you were single. Or to thank your lucky planets and other astrology stuff I don't understand that you already are.

Lucky 13-Minute Single Double Chocolate Chip Cookie

This cookie recipe came out of my desire, I'm sorry: my *desperate need*, for one cookie, instead of a whole batch (which would undoubtedly result in eating half of said batch of cookies)! Yes, leftovers are the bestovers, but sometimes cookie leftovers are the bestovers at making pants difficult to squeeze into. Yet sometimes a chocolate cookie is just necessary. Consider it indulgence without overindulgence. And consider baking it whenever you need a little self-care and extra sweetness in your life.

MAKES 1 COOKIE

¼ cup almond flour (a.k.a. almond meal)

1½ teaspoons cacao powder or cocoa powder (see page 315)

⅛ teaspoon baking soda

Pinch of sea salt or pink salt

1 tablespoon chocolate chips

1 tablespoon maple syrup

1 teaspoon vanilla extract

1 tablespoon almond butter

1½ teaspoons almond milk

1. Preheat the oven (or toaster oven if you want to relive your Easy-Bake days) to 350°F. Line a baking sheet with parchment paper.
2. Mix all of the ingredients in their listed order in a small bowl.
3. Use a spoon and your fingers to form the batter into one big cookie on the prepared baking sheet.
4. Bake for 13 minutes.
5. Remove it from the oven and let it sit for a couple of minutes to harden up.
6. Love this cookie and love yourself.

Banana Ice Cream

Banana ice cream is decadence without dairy. Sweetness without unnatural sugar. And it takes about 1 minute to make. (And about 1 ingredient.) I can promise you this: Once you go banana [ice cream], you'll never go back [to crappy ice cream].

You're going to want to get in the habit of peeling and freezing ripe bananas. (Ripe = speckled.) This is not only an acceptable way to take up freezer space, but it's fantastic for not letting any bananas go to waste. I always have a bag of frozen bananas in my freezer, the same way I always have a spare tire in my trunk. I cut peeled, ripe bananas into halves before popping them into ziplock bags to freeze them (at least overnight).

SERVES 1 (BUT IF SHARING IS HOW YOU SHOW CARING, EASY TO DOUBLE OR TRIPLE)

1½ to 2 frozen ripe banana, sliced into thick chunks

Other flavorings (optional; see below)

1. Add the banana chunks to a food processor and pulse about 15 times. (Scrape down the sides if the bananas start creeping up.)
2. Add any flavorings (optional). Pulse to incorporate.
3. Puree until just smooth and creamy.
4. No judgment for eating right out of the food processor. Less dishes equals less stresses.

Banana Ice Cream flavors on fleek!

Add to the base recipe:

Mint Chocolate Chip = Add 2 packed tablespoons fresh mint and process with the bananas, then stir in 2 tablespoons chocolate chips.

Strawberry = Add ¼ cup fresh or frozen strawberries, ¼ teaspoon vanilla extract, and a splash of almond milk and process with the bananas.

Matcha Coconut = After processing into ice cream, add 1 teaspoon matcha powder and process again, then stir in 2 tablespoons shredded coconut.

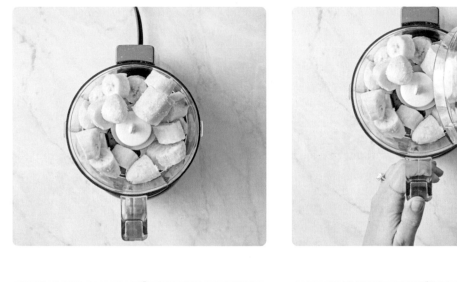

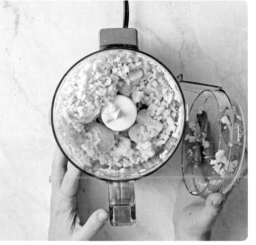

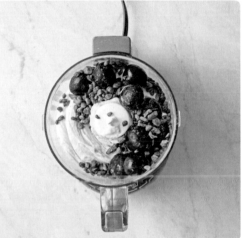

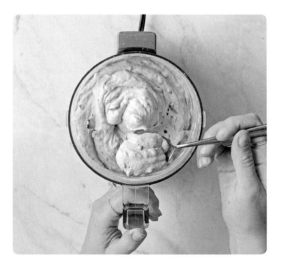

LEFTOVERS ARE THE BESTOVERS:

Banana Ice Cream doesn't actually freeze well, so in this case try to make only what you'll eat, or find a neighbor (or puppy if you didn't add chocolate) to help you out.

Chocolate Chocolate Chip = After processing into ice cream, add 1 tablespoon cocoa or cacao powder and a small pinch of sea salt and process again, then stir in 1 to 2 tablespoons of chocolate chips.

Peanut Butter Cup = After processing into ice cream, either add 1 to 2 peanut butter cups or stir in 1 to 2 tablespoons of peanut butter or almond butter, 1 to 2 tablespoons of chocolate chips, and a sprinkle of cinnamon.

Pumpkin Pie = After processing into ice cream, add ¼ cup pumpkin puree plus 1 teaspoon pumpkin pie spice and process again.

Chocolate Chip Cookie Dough = After processing into ice cream, add 1 to 2 Edible Chocolate Chip Cookie Dough balls (page 132), broken into bites.

Cherry Chocolate Chip (pictured on page 111) = Add ¼ cup frozen cherries to the frozen bananas for processing. Process until creamy, then add ¼ to ½ teaspoon vanilla extract or vanilla bean and process again. Stir in an additional 1 to 2 tablespoons of chocolate chips.

Salted Caramel = After processing into ice cream, stir in 2 tablespoons Caramel Fit for a Date (page 188) and top with a sprinkle of sea or pink salt.

Chocolate Fudge Brownie = After processing into ice cream, add in 1 tablespoon of cocoa or cacao powder and process again, then top with a leftover Fooled Ya Black Bean Brownie (page 279) and drizzle with the "Sexy Can I Drizzle This Magic Chocolate Sauce" (page 79).

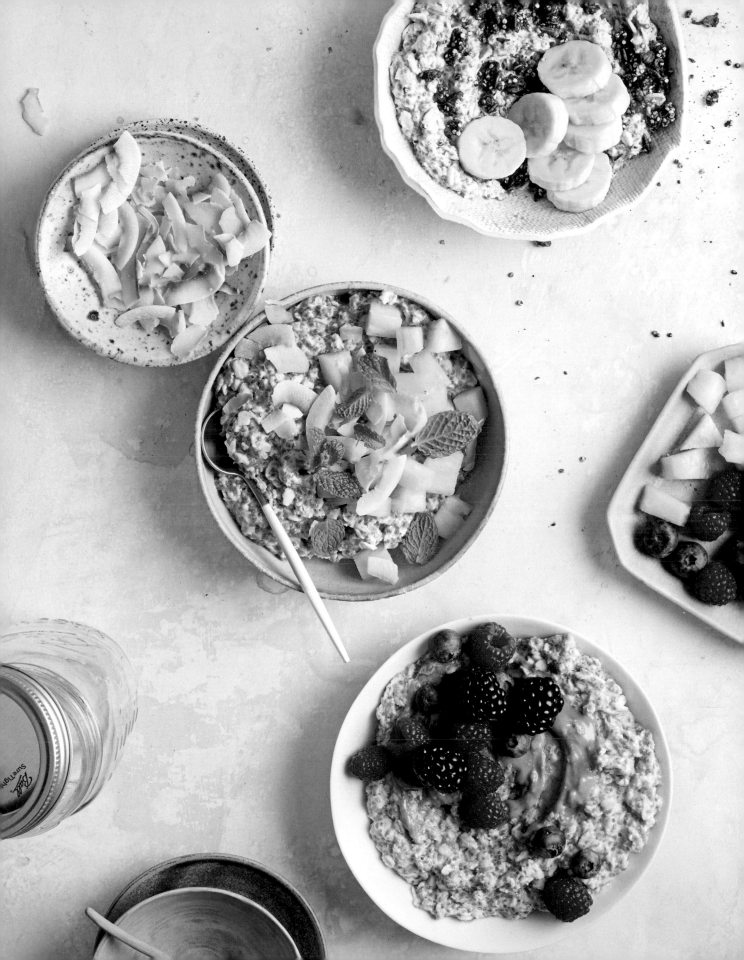

Chocolate = A responsible amount of "Sexy Can I Drizzle This Magic Chocolate Sauce" (page 79) and cacao nibs.

Tropical = 2 tablespoons coconut flakes and chopped pineapple and/or mango.

Before making your oats . . .

Matcha Muscles = Blend 2 tablespoons of your favorite plant-protein powder and 1 teaspoon of matcha into the almond milk and then continue to make your oats with your now-jacked-up milk.

Grab and BurritGOs!

I know jealousy is a bad look, but it inspired this fantastic breakfast, so it has its uses. In short, I was jealous of Jesse's ability to defrost sausage-stuffed breakfast sandwiches when I was stuck making my own morning glory from scratch. So one day I threw some of my tofu scramble in a wrap and froze it. Turns out, plant partiers can defrost yummy things, too, mofo! And then it was *his* turn to get green with envy.

MAKES 3 TO 4 BURRITOS

1 recipe Tofu Scramble de Talia (page 185)

1 15-ounce can black beans, drained and rinsed

4 large tortillas, whole-grain, spelt, brown-rice, and/or gluten-free as preferred

1. Prepare the Tofu Scramble de Talia with an additional drained and rinsed can of black beans, sautéed with the veggies. Allow to cool.
2. Scoop some of the tofu filling and place in the center of a tortilla. Fold in the edges, then roll up. Wrap in foil.
3. Repeat until filling is gone.
4. Store BurritGOs in the fridge or freezer. When you're ready to enjoy one, defrost it in the oven at 350°F for 15 minutes and then grab . . . and go!

WHEN YOU WORKED ALL DAY BUT STILL NEED TO COOK YOURSELF A QUICK DINNER BECAUSE LIFE SUCKS SOMETIMES

Once, on my podcast, I shamefully admitted to an organizational expert that I was so lazy that when I finished a toilet paper roll, I often just put the new one on *top* of the old one rather than replace it. She very kindly told me to open up the stopwatch—I mean phone timer, what's a stopwatch?—and time how long it actually took to replace the toilet paper roll. By the time I pressed go, the roll was already replaced.

Our perception of time can cockblock our healthy habits. Time yourself making these two dinners. Once you see how quick they are, you won't *not* be able to make them on those nights when you're burned-out but still need a super supper.

Staples R US Tahini TeriyakYAY Bowl

SERVES 3 TO 4

RICE

1 cup short-grain brown rice (2 cups if you're making this for many hungry humans), or 1 recipe Really Nice Cauliflower Rice (page 94)

SAUCE

2 tablespoons tahini

¼ cup tamari

½ teaspoon dried ginger

½ teaspoon garlic powder

1 tablespoon agave, maple syrup, or brown rice syrup

DISH

Fresh or frozen kale, quantity to preference, washed and chopped

Frozen edamame, quantity to preference

Frozen broccoli, quantity to preference

Frozen other veggie (cauliflower, mushrooms, carrots), quantity to preference

1 recipe of Sweet-Ass Sriracha Tofu (page 50)

1. Get your rice cooking, or make cauliflower rice. If making rice, place it in a pot on the stove. Add 2 cups water (4 cups if you're making this for many hungry humans), cover, and bring to a boil. When it's bubbling, reduce the heat to low and simmer as slowly as possible until all of the water has evaporated. Or make Really Nice Cauliflower Rice.

2. While it's cooking, whisk the tahini, tamari, ginger, garlic, and agave together in a small bowl. (Easy to double or triple as needed.) Set aside.

3. Add a steamer basket to a large pot and add water just until it touches the steamer basket.

4. Put the pot on the stove over high heat and cover it. When the water starts boiling and you see steam, add the frozen veggies and then the fresh veggies.

5. Steam for 5 minutes, or until they're your desired texture.

6. Assemble: In individual bowls, combine the cooked rice, some sauce, some veggies, and some Sweet-Ass Sriracha Tofu. Enjoy this take-out fake-out.

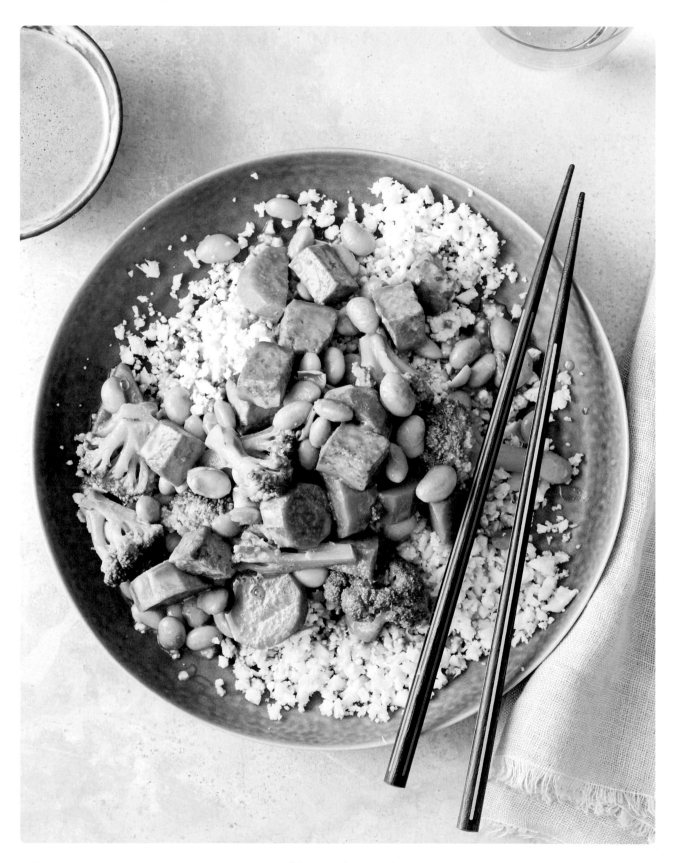

Tahini TeriyakYAY Bowl

Crazy-Quick Fettuccine Caulifredo Spaghetti Squasho

SERVES 3 TO 4

DISH

1 large spaghetti squash

2 teaspoons olive oil

Pink salt or sea salt and freshly ground pepper to taste

CAULIFREDO SAUCE

1 14.4-ounce bag frozen cauliflower florets

¾ cup plain, unsweetened almond milk or other nondairy milk, plus more as needed

1 tablespoon olive oil or vegan butter

2 large garlic cloves, minced

¼ cup nutritional yeast

¼ cup raw cashews, plus more as needed

Juice of ½ lemon

1 teaspoon pink salt or sea salt

Freshly ground black pepper to taste

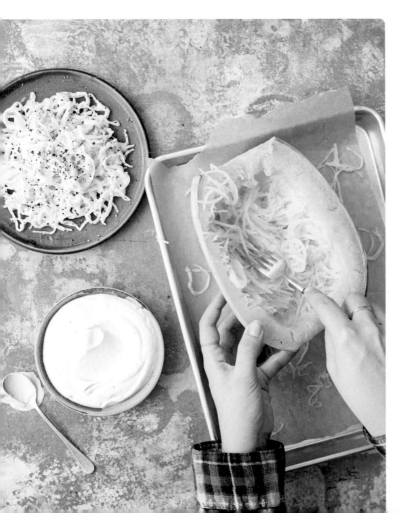

1. Preheat the oven to 400°F. Slice the ends off the squash and carefully cut the squash in half lengthwise.
2. Use a spoon (a grapefruit spoon would be superb if you have one) to scrape out and discard the seeds.
3. Drizzle 1 teaspoon of olive oil on each half of the squash and season generously with salt and pepper.
4. Lay the squash halves on a baking sheet facedown and bake for about 45 minutes (the squash is done when you press the upper skin and it's soft).
5. Remove the squash from the oven and let it cool for 10 minutes. Then use a fork to scrape out the inner part, revealing the magical spaghetti noodles.

6. While the squash cools, make the caulifredo sauce: Empty the bag of cauliflower into a large pot and add enough water to cover it plus an inch or two. Put it on the stove, cover with a lid, and bring to a boil.

7. Let it boil for 5 to 8 minutes. When a fork goes through the florets easily, it's done.

8. While it's cooking, place olive oil in a small saucepan over medium to high heat and add the garlic. Sauté for about 5 minutes, until the garlic is fragrant. Set aside.

9. Drain the cauliflower and add to a blender. Add the almond milk, oil, garlic, nutritional yeast, cashews, lemon juice, salt, and pepper.

10. Blend, baby, until super creamy and awesome. Add another splash of almond milk if you want it creamier or more cashews if you want it thicker.

11. Transfer the noodles to a bowl and smother with a generous amount of Caulifredo Sauce.

LEFTOVERS ARE THE BESTOVERS:

This sauce saves b-e-a-uuuutifully in a glass jar in your fridge. And in a stroke of good luck, spaghetti squash also saves s-p-e-c-t-aaaacularly. Put them together for an easy lunch mañana.

AFTER [PARTY] THOUGHT:

This dish is a layup for adding roasted or defrosted frozen peas, broccoli, asparagus, or other greens. Drizzle your veggie with olive oil and salt and pepper and roast it in the parameters of the pan.

WHEN YOU'RE COZILY READING A BOOK IN A NOOK, OR DOING ANYTHING IN SLIPPERS

When I asked my recipe testers if they thought I'd covered every situation in their daily lives, my buddy Madeline asked where the dish for "cozily reading a book in a nook" was. I wondered how she *had* a reading nook and then I remembered that I live in New York City and she's in Colorado. So I sat on my dog's bed—my new reading nook!—and dreamed up this cozy and nutritious chai banana bread that goes perfectly with homemade hot chocolate and a good book. Or a good Kindle. Or a good pair of head-phones (for an audiobook[8]). PSA: These recipes also work if you're cud-dling with a human or canine instead of a book.

ZZZ^z

8 Or a podcast! Like my *Party in My Plants* podcast ayoo!

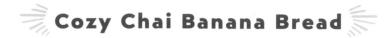

Cozy Chai Banana Bread

MAKES 1 LOAF (6 TO 10 SLICES)

2 tablespoons flax meal (or use 2 regular eggs if you eat 'em)

2 cups mashed super ripe bananas (3 to 4 brown speckled ones)

⅓ cup maple syrup

1 teaspoon vanilla extract

¼ cup melted refined coconut oil (if you can find butter-flavored coconut oil, it would be perfect in this recipe)

2 tablespoons almond milk

2 cups spelt flour (whole-wheat or all-purpose gluten-free flour works, too)

1 teaspoon baking soda

1 tablespoon cinnamon

1 teaspoon cardamom

2 teaspoons allspice

1 teaspoon dried ginger

½ teaspoon sea salt or pink salt

½ teaspoon nutmeg

2 tablespoons coconut sugar

¼ to ½ cup chopped raw walnuts (optional)

1. Preheat the oven to 350°F. Line a 9 x 5-inch loaf pan with parchment paper or spray it with coconut oil.
2. Make the flax eggs by combining the flax meal and 6 tablespoons water in a small bowl or cup, stir with a fork, and set aside.
3. Place the flour, baking soda, cinnamon, cardamom, allspice, ginger, salt, nutmeg, and coconut sugar in a large mixing bowl.
4. When the flax eggs are gooey and the water has bonded to the flax meal, combine the flax eggs, bananas, maple syrup, vanilla, coconut oil, and almond milk in a medium bowl and mix together.
5. Combine the wet ingredients with the dry ingredients in the larger mixing bowl and stir to combine. No dry portions left behind!
6. Stir in the nuts if you're using them.
7. Pour your batter into the prepared loaf pan. Spread it out so it'll bake evenly.

8. Bake for 55 minutes, or until a small knife or toothpick comes out clean.

9. Let it cool. Store leftovers covered in the fridge.

LEFTOVERS ARE THE BESTOVERS:

Heat a slice up for breakfast in your toaster oven and top it with a drizzle of maple syrup, nut butter, or Caramel Fit for a Date (page 188).

AFTER [PARTY] THOUGHT:

Transform this recipe into a dreamy pumpkin bread. Use canned pumpkin instead of mashed banana; lose the cardamom, allspice, and nutmeg; add 1 tablespoon of pumpkin pie spice and ¼ teaspoon of ground cloves; and adjust the cinnamon to 1½ teaspoons and ginger to ¼ teaspoon. Mix in ¼ to ½ cup chocolate chips and/or ¼ to ½ cup pecan pieces instead of walnuts (optional).

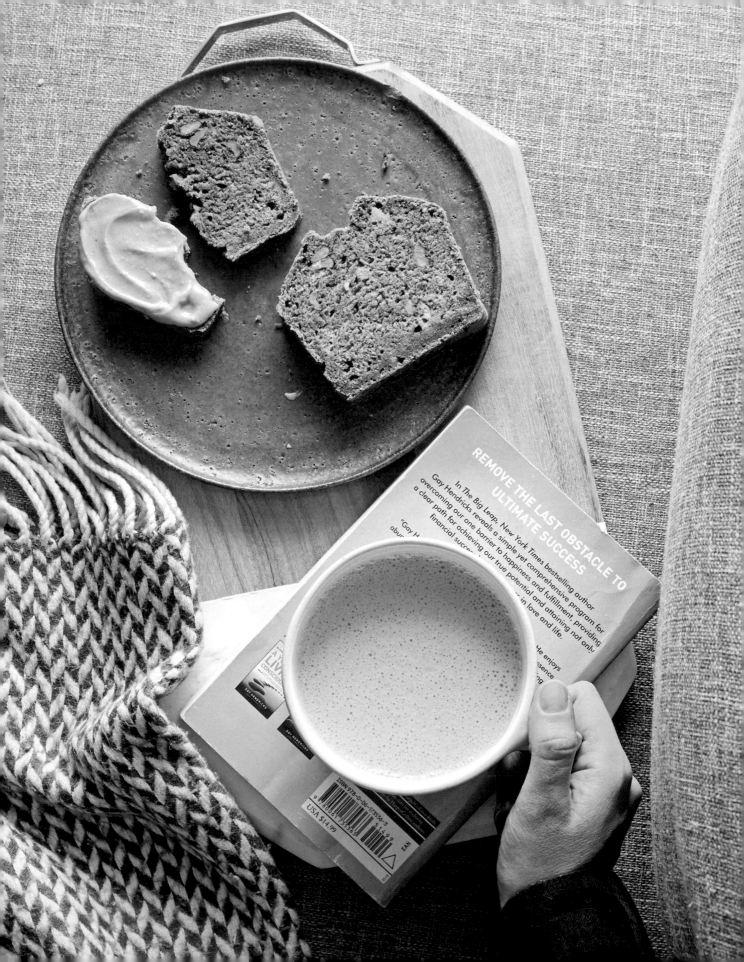

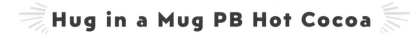

Hug in a Mug PB Hot Cocoa

MAKES 1 MUG FULL

1½ cups almond milk or other unsweetened plant milk

1 tablespoon cacao or cocoa powder

1 to 2 tablespoons peanut butter, almond butter, or tahini

½ teaspoon vanilla extract

⅛ teaspoon cinnamon

1 Medjool date or 1 to 2 teaspoons coconut sugar, organic cane sugar, palm sugar, honey, maple syrup, or stevia to taste

1. Add the almond milk, cacao powder, peanut butter, vanilla, cinnamon, and date to blender and blend until frothy. If you have a Vitamix, just leave it on high for a few minutes and it'll heat itself. If not, pour this frothy goodness into a small pot on the stove over medium to medium-high heat and warm it to your desired temperature. I like to bring it to a light boil and then immediately remove it from the heat.

2. Pour into a mug and sip.

NOTE: If using a date, soak it in warm water for at least 10 minutes to soften before blending.

Cozy Chai Banana Bread with Hug in a Mug PB Hot Cocoa

WHEN YOU HAD A BAD DAY

After a really lousy day, sometimes a long bath is all we need to feel better, or a chat with our bestie. Other times, a good scream into our pillow does the trick. Or a good sob in your car or Uber. But there are times where the only solution is to cry . . . into some comfort food. The magic is making sure you're crying into the *right* comfort food—the stuff that won't make you feel worse in the morning. Which happens to be this plant-packed Quesa[BAD DAY]dilla, which couldn't be comfort foodier, and this Edible Chocolate Chip Cookie Dough (page 132) that tastes similar to the cheer-me-up salmonella stuff without the risk of, well, salmonella.

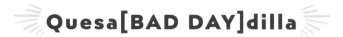

Quesa[BAD DAY]dilla

SERVES 2 (DOUBLE, TRIPLE, OR HALVE AS NEEDED)

GUAC-ISH

1 ripe avocado

Juice of ½ lime

¼ to ½ teaspoon sea salt or pink salt

Fresh cilantro to taste

QUESADILLA

1 sweet potato (peeled if not organic), chopped into flat or thin chunks

Half of an 8-ounce package of tempeh, coarsely chopped (optional, but optimal for added protein)

1 cup spinach

2 large tortillas per person, made from rice flour, spelt, or whatever you like

½ 16-ounce can of refried pinto beans (refried black beans work, too)

2 cups shredded dairy-free or goat cheese

Coconut oil or olive oil for sautéing

1 cup salsa

Hot sauce to taste

1. Make the Guac-ish (because it's the easiest guac I feel weird even calling it guacamole). Smash the flesh from the avocado in a bowl with a fork. Add the lime juice, salt, and cilantro if using (if your other half hates cilantro, like Jesse does, leave it on the side). Set aside.

2. In a medium to large pot, add a steamer basket and sprawl it out. Fill the pot with enough water so it just about becomes visible through the steamer basket. Cover the pot, put it on the stove over high heat, and bring the water to a boil.

3. Add the sweet potato chunks, reduce the heat, and cover again. Steam for 3 to 5 minutes. Add the tempeh chunks if using, and steam for another 4 minutes. Finally, add the spinach and steam for 2 to 3 minutes, or until it wilts. Remove from the heat and take everything out of the pot with tongs.

4. Assemble the quesadillas by spreading one tortilla out on a large plate or cutting board and adding the pinto or black beans on top, leaving about ½ inch of room on the sides like a pizza crust.

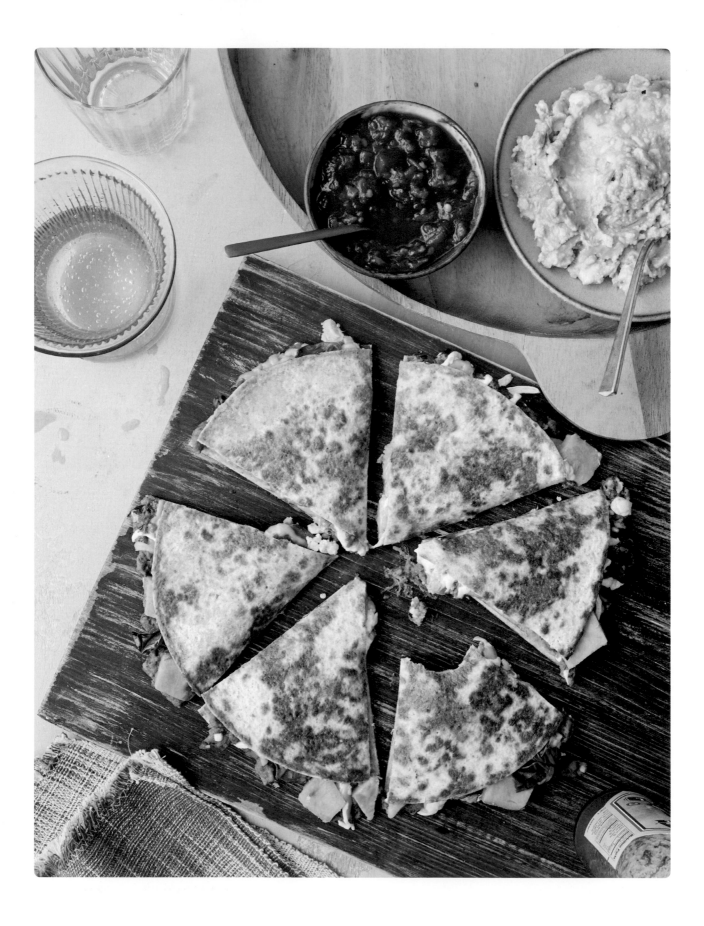

5. Use your fingers to crumble the tempeh on top of the beans.

6. Sprinkle on a hefty amount of your preferred cheese, the sweet potatoes, and the wilted spinach. Add another light dusting of cheese to serve as glue and top with another tortilla.

7. Carry your plate with the quesadilla to the stove and heat the coconut oil in a large skillet or griddle over medium heat. Add the quesadilla. Cook for 3 to 4 minutes, until the bottom tortilla is lightly browned. Then use a spatula and the power of positive thinking to flip and cook the other side for 3 to 4 minutes, until it's also a little tan.

8. Remove from the heat. Use a serrated knife to slice it into four (or more) wedges, and serve with an abundance of salsa, Guac-ish, and hot sauce.

LEFTOVERS ARE THE BESTOVERS:

Make a quick breakfast by adding a scrambled egg or tofu.
Just some food for early a.m. thought.

 NOTE: Freaked out about awful flipping skills? Consider baking your 'dillas instead, at 375°F for 5 minutes, and then broil it for 2 minutes or until the cheese melts.

Edible Chocolate Chip Cookie Dough

SERVES 6 . . . ISH

1 15-ounce can chickpeas, drained and rinsed

½ cup almond butter or other nut or seed butter

¼ cup maple syrup

½ teaspoon cinnamon

2 teaspoons vanilla extract

¼ teaspoon salt

2 tablespoons rolled oats

Chocolate chips, as many as you need

1. Place the chickpeas, almond butter, maple syrup, cinnamon, vanilla, salt, and rolled oats in a food processor and process together.
2. Stir in the chocolate chips.
3. Eat with a spoon.

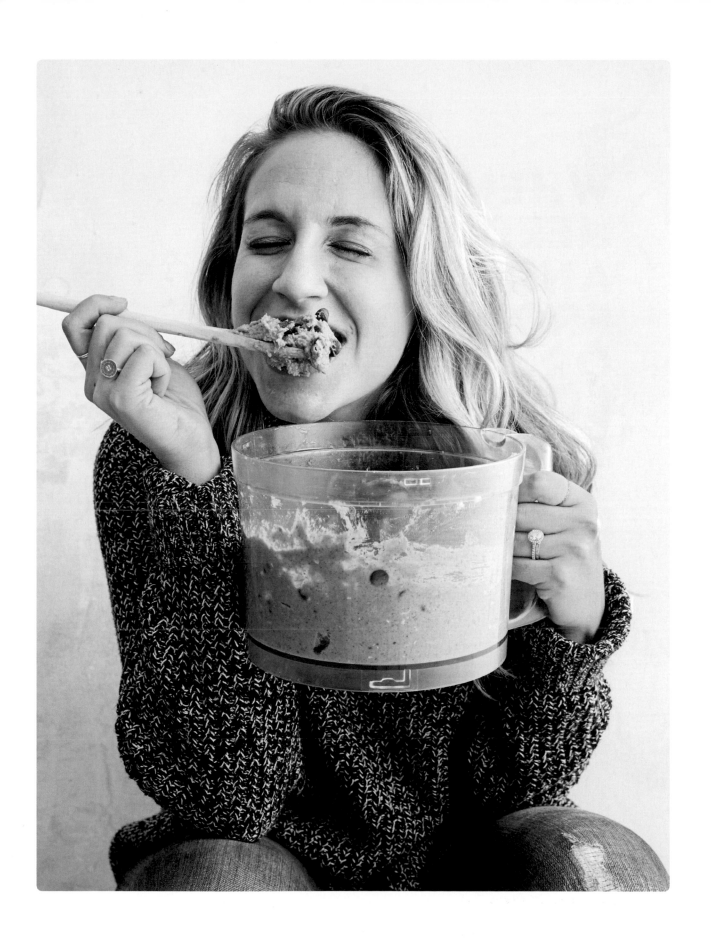

WHEN YOU NEED LUNCH AND YOU WORK FROM HOME OR YOU BRING LUNCH TO WORK

I'm the daughter of two parents who worked from home. They left me with no chance of getting a real job after growing up not watching my dad go off to work with a suit and briefcase but rather saunter into his office in a bathrobe. Like father, like daughter, because most days the clock strikes 2:00 p.m. and I'm stoked if I've brushed my teeth. It's taken me years to master actually making lunch when I'm working from home, so I'm proud as can be to present my No-Pants Salad, which uses fridge mainstays, takes max six minutes, requires zero chopping, and often gets eaten in my typical office attire: pants-less.

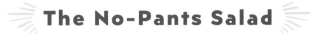

The No-Pants Salad

SERVES 1

3 large handfuls of arugula or mesclun salad mix

½ to ¾ cup cooked leftover quinoa (method on page 96)

2 tablespoons raw pumpkin seeds (if you have them)

1 to 2 handfuls of sprouts (if you have them)

Shredded pecorino cheese, crumbled goat cheese, nutritional yeast, or shredded vegan cheese to taste

2 forkfuls of raw sauerkraut

Protein of your choice—a chopped-up veggie burger, leftover lentils, leftover tofu or tempeh, or white, black, or other beans from a can, drained and rinsed

Your Greens' New Go-To DRESSing (page 213) to taste

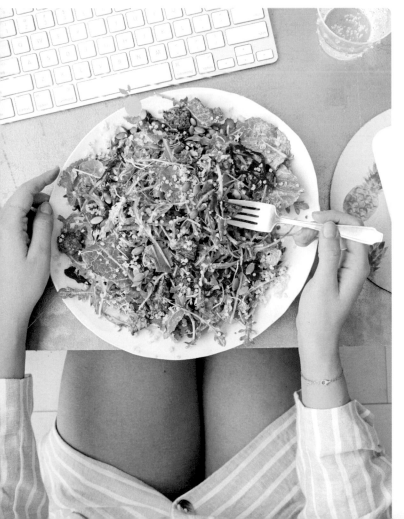

1. Combine the arugula, quinoa, pumpkin seeds, sprouts, cheese, sauerkraut, protein, and dressing in a large bowl and toss.

2. Sit! Eat! Away from your computer.

3. Then, get back to work.

WHEN YOU'RE ENTERTAINING, OR GOING SOMEWHERE TO BE ENTERTAINED

I pride myself on being a low-key entertainee. I, Your Honor, need not much to have a good time.

Because I bring it all myself.

Whether it's a Fourth of July cookout, a ten-person dinner party, or a meet-my-new-baby brunch, my rule of thumb is: Do not expect a plant party awaiting, so bring the plant party yourself. The cool thing about taking care of yourself is that when you bring goodies, you come off looking like an incredibly generous guest. Win-win.

THE TWO OR THREE THINGS TO BRING TO EVERY AFFAIR:
1) a hearty protein-based dish, 2) a dessert, and 3) kombucha.

Hearty plant party because you'll likely have no protein options to fill you up. Most salads and veggie sides at these junctions are the reasons people think healthy eating sucks in the first place.

Dessert because the worst thing in the world is not being able to eat dessert. (The only thing worse is eating dessert that makes you feel like crap.) They are the easiest to make, they give you an opportunity to prove how healthy food can be even yummier than the other stuff on offer (which usually leads to you stealing the show and pranking everyone with the big reveal that the dish they're swooning over is both delicious *and* nutritious).

Kombucha because it mixes perfectly with light spirits or perfectly takes the place of light spirits. (See Our 'Bucha Mule on page 155.)

Thoughts on Entertaining, or
Going Somewhere to Be Entertained

My best friend's mom is a tray lady, meaning that for twenty-five years, I've watched her fill trays with little bowls for snacking. Whether we were watching *Rugrats*, weighing pros and cons of colleges, or planning my wedding, as long as we were near Cyral, we'd be near a tray of assorted snacks. (And when I had my said wedding, guess what her gift was?) But it took me until age thirty to fully appreciate a tray's magnificence. What better way to make someone happily sit and stay for a while than by shoving a medley of nourishing nibbles in front of their face? Here are some of my favorite things to put on one of my now-many trays.

Eggplant Fries (+ Special Sauce)

Eggplant being underrated is an understatement, but it took me a while to get the memo. Since it's a nightshade niece of the best frying plant (potato), it should be no surprise that this is one purple people pleaser.

SERVES 3 TO 4 AS A SIDE

1 large eggplant

2 tablespoons olive oil

1 teaspoon sea salt or pink salt

½ teaspoon freshly ground black pepper

1 teaspoon smoked or sweet paprika

2 teaspoon maple syrup

¾ cup almond meal or flour (or oat or rice flour if allergic to nuts)

2 tablespoons nutritional yeast

Special Sauce (recipe follows)

1. Preheat the oven to 400°F. Line a rimmed baking sheet with parchment paper.
2. Wash and dry the eggplant and then cut it into thin, fry-like sticks. (The thinner they are, the crispier they will get.)
3. Place the eggplant fries in a large bowl and sprinkle with the olive oil. Toss around to coat every fry.
4. Add the salt, pepper, paprika, and maple syrup. Toss again to coat every fry with the goods.
5. Add the almond meal and nutritional yeast and, again, toss the fries to coat them well.
6. Spread the fries out on the baking sheet and slide the baking sheet into the oven.
7. Bake for about 45 minutes, or until golden brown. While they're baking, make the sauce.
8. Store any leftovers (yeah, right) sealed in the fridge. They're equally delightful reheated in the oven or eaten cold.

continued

NOTE: In lieu of an oven you can use an air fryer. Hey, if you've got it—flaunt and fry in it. And give it a few good shakes in the air fryer now and then to make sure all the fries get nice and golden. (Thanks, BL!)

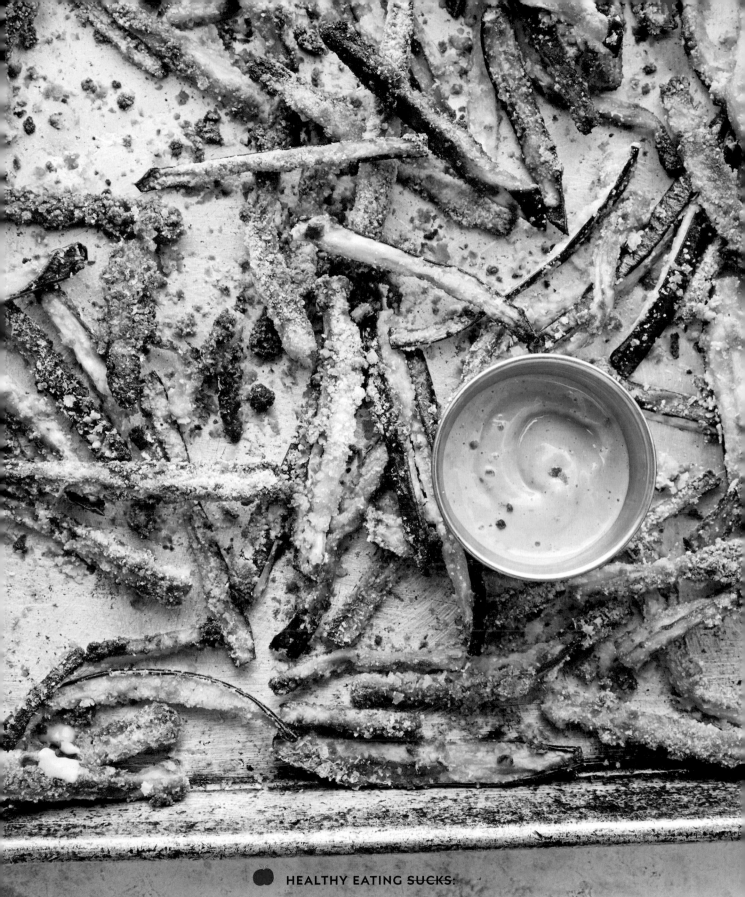

"I didn't think I liked eggplant until this recipe. Talia, you completely opened my mind!" —AS

AFTER [PARTY] THOUGHT:

Throwing shade on nightshades? If you're avoiding tomatoes, white potatoes, peppers, and eggplant for autoimmune reasons, use zucchini instead.

LEFTOVERS ARE THE BESTOVERS:

This makes a lot, which is favorable because of the whole "make any, many many" thing. Leftovers go nicely on baked sweet potatoes (or Sweet Potato Wedgies on page 97)—or, of course, more eggplant or zucchini fries. You can also drizzle with tahini and pomegranate seeds and serve 'em cold.

SERVE WITH THIS QUICK SPECIAL SAUCE:

1 14-ounce package of soft or silken tofu, drained

2 tablespoons sriracha (3 tablespoons if you like it really spicy)

¼ cup ketchup

2 tablespoons coconut sugar

1 teaspoon sea salt or pink salt

½ teaspoon apple cider vinegar

Add the tofu, ketchup, coconut sugar, salt, and apple cider vinegar to a blender and blend until smooth.

Better Than a Snickers Bar Bites

These bites come off wildly impressive (despite being wildly easy), and really, they're always a good idea. The only time they'd be a bad idea is if a nut-allergic person wants to eat them—in which case you can substitute sunflower butter or tahini, which makes you a super-considerate and all-inclusive superhero.

MAKES 12 TO 16 BITES

½ cup chocolate chips, your desired darkness

1 teaspoon refined coconut oil

Pinch of sea salt

1 to 2 tablespoons crunchy or smooth peanut butter for the chocolate mixture, plus more peanut butter to taste

12 Medjool dates, pitted

Crushed peanut pieces or crumbs, shredded coconut, cacao nibs, or sprinkles to taste

1. Line a plate with parchment papter. Using a double boiler or a microwave, melt the chocolate with the coconut oil.

2. Mix in the salt and peanut butter and combine until smooth.

3. One at a time, use a knife to stuff each date with the nut butter. Fold the date back together and roll it in the melted chocolate mixture so it's completely covered.

4. Use the wet chocolate covering the dates as "glue" and roll the dates in (or sprinkle the top with) crushed peanut pieces or crumbs, shredded coconut, cacao nibs, or sprinkles.

5. Place on the parchment–lined plate.

6. Repeat until all the chocolate is gone.

7. Freeze the dates for 10 to 15 minutes, remove from the freezer, and enjoy. You can also store them for later, as these guys are great right out of the fridge or freezer for those nights you MUST have dessert or the world will end.

HEALTHY EATING SUCKS:

"My boyfriend loved them. He hates dates and didn't even realize it was a date until after he ate it."

—CS

WHAT TO MAKE WHEN, GO SHORTY!, IT'S YOUR BIRTHDAY! OR SOMEONE ELSE'S BIRTHDAY, OR ANYONE ON FACEBOOK'S BIRTHDAY

My love for Funfetti cupcakes runs deep. I mean, it literally contains the word "fun." My lucky mother got so much praise in my youth because I thought she *invented* them. I've noticed that being a health-conscious grown-up means that Funfetti cupcakes aren't as much of a thing, and birthdays are less fun because of it. My versions still have sprinkles but don't lead to bloat, blood sugar spikes, or bellyaches. So you know how they say "Every party need a pooper?" Well, that pooper is whoever finishes the last Less-Unhealthy Funfetti Cupcake (page 144)!

Less-Unhealthy Funfetti Cupcakes

VANILLA VERSION

Dry Ingredients

2½ cups spelt flour (or a gluten-free mix 1:1, such as Bob's Red Mill)

1 teaspoon baking powder

1 teaspoon baking soda

2 pinches of sea salt

¼ cup coconut sugar or organic cane sugar

Sprinkles (optional)

Wet Ingredients

1 cup almond milk, unsweetened

½ cup melted coconut oil (butter flavored if you can find it)

½ cup maple syrup

¼ cup unsweetened applesauce

2 teaspoons apple cider vinegar

1 teaspoon vanilla extract

½ teaspoon lemon extract (optional)

CHOCOLATE VERSION

Dry Ingredients

2½ cups spelt flour (or a gluten-free mix 1:1, such as Bob's Red Mill)

¼ cup cacao or cocoa powder

1 teaspoon baking powder

1 teaspoon baking soda

2 pinches of sea salt

¼ cup coconut sugar or organic cane sugar

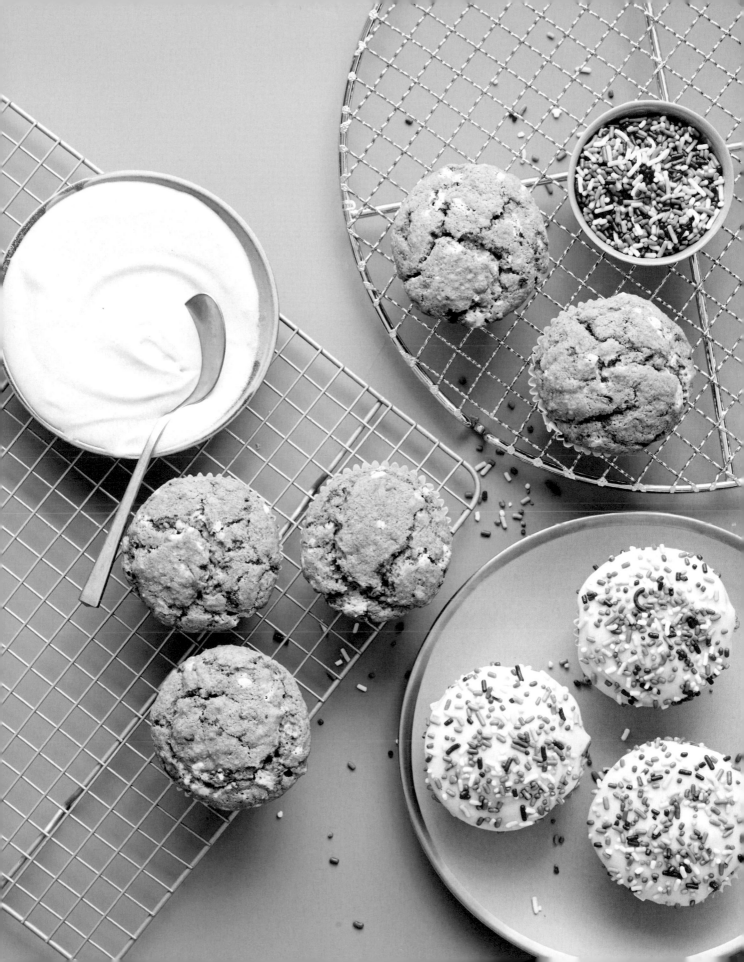

Wet Ingredients

1 cup almond milk, unsweetened

½ cup melted coconut oil (even better if it's butter-flavored)

½ cup maple syrup or honey

¼ cup unsweetened applesauce

2 teaspoons apple cider vinegar

1 teaspoon vanilla extract

1 cup chocolate chips

Sprinkles (optional)

1. Preheat the oven to 350°F. Line a muffin tin with cupcake liners.
2. Mix the dry ingredients in a bowl.
3. Mix the wet ingredients in another bowl.
4. Mix the wet ingredients into the dry ingredients.
5. Add sprinkles and mix to incorporate.
6. Divide the batter equally to fill each muffin cup three-quarters to the top.
7. Bake for 20 minutes for full-size cupcakes or about 17 minutes if you're making mini cupcakes. They're done when you slide a toothpick into them and it slides out clean! Or when you touch the top of them with your finger and it doesn't leave a permanent indent.
8. Remove from the oven and let cool.
9. Spread the frosting (recipe follows) on top and immediately sprinkle with additional sprinkles if using.
10. Store leftovers in a sealed container in the fridge.

CRAP-FREE VANILLA FROSTING

¾ cup raw cashews

¼ cup coconut yogurt

1 tablespoon coconut oil, melted

½ teaspoon vanilla extract

3 to 5 tablespoons maple syrup

Pinch of sea salt

1. Soak the cashews in water for at least 1 hour—the longer the better.
2. Drain and rinse the cashews and place in a blender along with all of the other ingredients.
3. Blend until creamy.
4. Transfer to a glass jar and let chill in the fridge until it's thick like frosting, about 10 minutes.

CRAP-FREE CHOCOLATE FROSTING

1 cup coconut milk (full-fat from a can)

1¼ cups chocolate chips

1 teaspoon coconut oil

½ teaspoon vanilla extract

2 tablespoons maple syrup or honey

Pinch of salt

1. Heat the coconut milk in a saucepan until it's just starting to simmer.
2. Place the chocolate chips in a heatproof bowl (not plastic).
3. Pour the hot coconut milk over the chocolate chips and stir/whisk to melt.
4. Add the coconut oil (which doesn't have to be soft because it'll melt), vanilla, maple syrup, and salt and whisk.
5. Either place the whole bowl in the fridge or move the frosting to a glass jar and let that chill in the fridge until it hardens to a spreadable texture, about 40 minutes.

HEALTHY EATING SUCKS:

"My husband ate these and then sent me a gif of
Homer Simpson drooling. Soooooo, success!"

—MD

WHEN IT'S TOO DAMN HOT BUT YOU STILL GOTTA EAT

When the idea of coming within a five-foot radius of an oven can put you in an extra-hot sweat, slurping down a smoothie can be a midsummer night's (and day's) (and afternoon's) dream. But sometimes you want something that requires more than a straw (if they're still legal at the time of printing this book) or a glass rim. That's where Watermelon Gazpacho, which is basically just a chilly soupy salad, saves the day. Follow it up with this Banana Cream Pie (page 150), which is so good it might be worth cranking the heat and blasting reggae for all year-round. Speaking from experience.

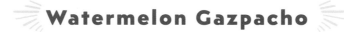

Watermelon Gazpacho

2 cups watermelon chunks

1 tablespoon freshly squeezed lime juice (juice from about ½ lime)

1 medium tomato

1 tablespoon chopped fresh basil

1 tablespoon chopped fresh mint

½ teaspoon minced ginger

½ teaspoon chopped jalapeño (optional)

1 garlic clove

2 pinches of sea salt

½ cup chopped tomato

½ cup chopped cucumber

Basil, chopped and to taste, for garnish

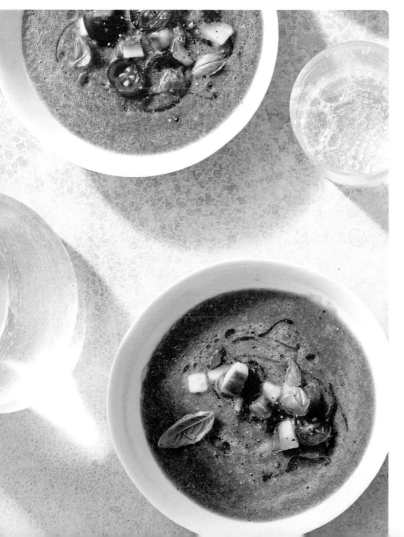

1. Blend together 1½ cups of watermelon chunks, the lime juice, tomato, basil, mint, ginger, jalapeño, if using, garlic, and salt.
2. Pour the soup into a large bowl and add the remaining ½ cup watermelon chunks, tomato, cucumber, and basil.
3. Mix everything together and dive in.

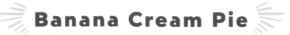

Banana Cream Pie

SERVES 6 TO 8

CRUST

1½ cups raw pecans, walnuts, or almonds

1½ cups pitted Medjool dates (give them a 10-minute warm water bath first)

2 pinches of salt

FILLING

1¼ cups raw cashews, soaked for at least 4 hours or overnight in a bowl with warm water, drained and rinsed

3 tablespoons refined coconut oil, melted

½ cup maple syrup or honey

½ cup full-fat coconut milk, ideally refrigerate overnight (open the can and just use ½ cup of the hardened creamy thick white part. You can blend the leftover cream and water from the can in smoothies throughout the week.)

1 teaspoon vanilla extract

¼ teaspoon sea salt or pink salt

2 to 3 tablespoons freshly squeezed lemon juice

2 very ripe bananas, mashed with a fork (about 1 cup mashed bananas)

GARNISHES

Creamy peanut butter to taste, plus more to drizzle (optional)

Chocolate chips (optional)

"Sexy Can I Drizzle This Magic Chocolate Sauce" (page 79) to taste (optional)

1. Do the prep work: The night before, put a can of full-fat coconut milk in the fridge and get the cashews soaking.

2. Make your crust: Process the nuts, dates, and salt together in a food processor until you can't recognize the nuts or the dates anymore. The dough should stick together and feel moldable. If it's too dry, add another date or two. If it's too wet, add a couple of extra nuts.

3. Press the dough into an 8- or 9-inch pie pan, round springform cake pan, or 8 x 8-inch baking dish. Make sure your crust fills the bottom and goes up a tiny bit on the sides of the dish. If you plan to serve it on a different plate, line the dish with parchment paper or plastic wrap for easy removal.

4. Put the crust in the freezer while you make the filling.

5. Blend all of the filling ingredients in a blender for 1 to 2 minutes until silky smooth.

6. Remove the pan with the crust from the freezer. Pour the filling into the crust. Use a spoon or spatula to spread evenly. Feel free to drizzle creamy peanut butter, sprinkle with chocolate chips, or top with chocolate sauce.

7. Freeze for at least 4 hours.

8. When you're ready to eat it, let it thaw for 5 to 10 minutes (if you can exercise such patience). Then either remove it from the pan and onto a serving plate using the parchment/plastic wrap or slice it right from the pan.

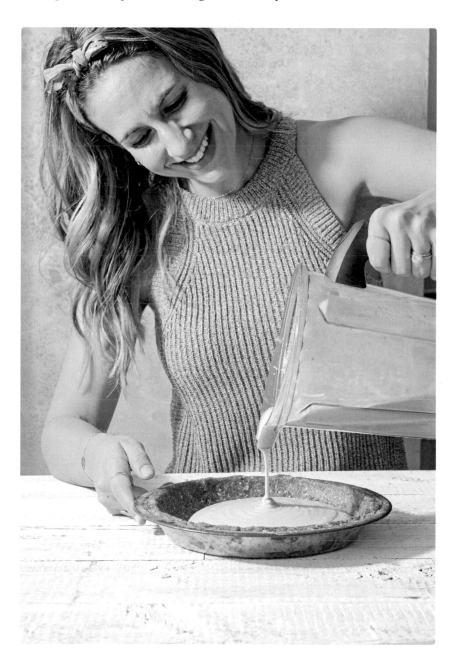

WHEN YOU'RE THROWING A DINNER PARTY WITH A TABLE RUNNER AND EVERYTHING

In the classic icebreaker Two Truths and a Lie, I always get people good by telling them that one of my favorite activities is cooking for other people. Truth: It's one of my biggest fears. Taste preferences are as personal as sexual ones and I worry that what pleases my buds won't tickle the fancy of all my buds' buds. But these recipes are tried and true and I confidently stand by them also pleasing you! So now I need a new lie for the game. Maybe that I can whistle?

Showstopping Stuffed Bell Peppers

I hate sharing food. Nothing brings me more pleasure than a non-shareable dish, which is exactly what this is. Give each person a pepper overflowing with protein-rich (thanks to quinoa and white beans), flavor-rich (thanks to tons of herbs, cheese, and spices) goodies—goodies they can hoard—and you've got the perfect dinner party.

SERVES 4

½ cup quinoa or brown rice

4 bell peppers

1 teaspoon finely ground sea salt or pink salt, plus a pinch

Pinch of freshly ground black pepper

Splash of coconut, avocado, or olive oil, plus olive oil to drizzle (optional)

2 garlic cloves, minced

½ yellow onion, chopped

1 can white beans (a.k.a. cannellini), drained and rinsed

¼ cup basil leaves, chopped fine (I use my mini food processor to chop all the herbs and seeds for me)

¼ cup parsley leaves, chopped fine

2 tablespoons pumpkin seeds, chopped fine (optional)

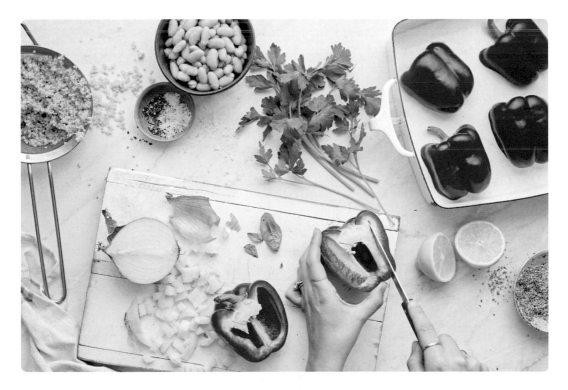

1 tablespoon freshly squeezed lemon juice (about ½ lemon)

2 heaping handfuls of spinach, chopped

½ cup goat, feta, or vegan cheese (¼ cup optional)

½ teaspoon dried oregano

1. Preheat the oven to 425°F. Line a rimmed baking sheet with parchment paper.
2. Cook the quinoa according to the package's instructions.
3. Cut the bell peppers in half lengthwise and remove the stems and seeds.
4. Place the bell peppers on the baking sheet, open-side down.
5. Bake for 15 minutes. Remove from the oven, flip so the open side is up, sprinkle with a pinch of salt and black pepper, and bake for another 15 minutes.
6. While the bell peppers are baking, prepare the filling: In a sauté pan over medium heat, add the coconut oil and cook the garlic and onion for 3 minutes.
7. Add the cooked quinoa, white beans, basil, parsley, pumpkin seeds, lemon juice, spinach, ¼ cup of the cheese, the remaining 1 teaspoon sea salt, and the oregano and sauté over medium-low to medium heat for 5 to 7 minutes, to heat everything thoroughly.
8. When the bell peppers are done, remove them from the oven and use a spoon to stuff each with the quinoa mix.
9. Drizzle the tops with olive oil if using, or top them with the remaining ¼ cup of crumbled cheese if using and switch your oven setting to broil for 3 to 4 minutes to get a crispy top.
10. Serve hot or at room temperature and store leftovers covered in the fridge.

LEFTOVERS ARE THE BESTOVERS:

These puppies heat up beautifully in the oven or microwave
for lunch the next day with tomato and cucumber or over greens.

OUR 'BUCHA MULE

Moscow Mules are kind of my family's "thing." Whenever we go on vacation, you better believe that on night one, you can find my dad unpacking his safely undie-and-sock-wrapped copper mugs in our rental house kitchen. Add to our traveling obsession with this gingery drink that this healthified Kombucha Mule was the signature drink at my wedding, I fully stand behind this being a true crowd pleaser. And considering it's made with great-for-your-gut ginger kombucha and not beer, I can stand by this being a belly pleaser to boot.

MAKES 1 DRINK (EASY TO DOUBLE OR EIGHT-LE)

6 ounces ginger kombucha

1 shot vodka (1½ ounces)

1 ounce freshly squeezed lime juice (about 1 lime)

1½ teaspoons agave (optional)

Mint leaf or lime wedge, for garnish

Ice

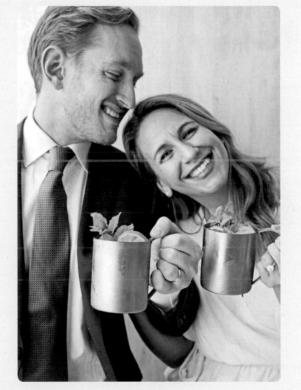

1. Combine the kombucha, vodka, lime juice, and agave, if using, and shake or stir over ice in a glass or jar. Garnish with mint.
2. Enjoy.

🍎 **HEALTHY EATING SUCKS:**

"My fiancé LOVED it. He said it's the only way he'll drink kombucha." —BM

Dr. Oz Said Everyone in America Should Be Eating This Kale Mint Chocolate Chip Ice Cream, So . . .

It was a random Tuesday night and I was in the kitchen making dinner with Jesse when I got a call from my favorite producer at *The Dr. Oz Show*: "Hi, we're doing a segment about what's new in kale. So, what's new in kale?" Caught off guard, I stammered and said, "Ummm, well, not kale chips . . . not kale salad . . ." as I tried to come up with something that would blow her mind. Jesse mouthed my favorite thing on the planet: "Ice cream?" So I said, "Kale ice cream?" The producer said, "Amazing. Love it. Have the recipe for me tomorrow." And that's how TV works. And that's how little time I had to trial and error this recipe from inedible (RIP batches 1, 2, and 3) into something that Dr. Oz said, while making direct eye contact with the camera lens, "everyone in America should be eating." He also called it orgasmic. And he's a doctor.

SERVES 6

1½ cups raw cashews

1½ cups nondairy milk

2 cups fresh kale, washed, rinsed, and torn into small pieces (I recommend the "dino" or "lacinato" variety, but curly kale works, too)

½ cup maple syrup, raw honey, or agave

1 tablespoon vanilla extract

2 teaspoons peppermint extract (optional; feel free to skip and just make chocolate chip ice cream)

Pinch of sea salt

2 tablespoons refined coconut oil, melted

4 tablespoons chocolate chips or mix-in of your choice (sprinkles, cookie crumbs, coconut flakes, etc.)

1. Add the cashews to a large bowl and cover with warm water. Set aside for at least 1 hour (even longer is even better).

2. Strain the water and rinse the cashews and then place the cashews in a blender.

3. Add the milk, kale, maple syrup, vanilla, peppermint extract, if using, and salt and blend until creamy.

4. Add the coconut oil and blend for another 5 to 10 seconds.

5. Transfer the mixture to a freezable container and stir in the chocolate chips.

6. Cover and let freeze for at least 6 hours or overnight.

7. Dive in with a spoon. If you have time to plan ahead, note that this ice cream's at its absolute creamy best when it's been left out to thaw for 1 hour plus.

AFTER [PARTY] THOUGHT:

Not into mint? Cut it out and add an extra teaspoon of vanilla instead.

HEALTHY EATING SUCKS:

"I just want to always have it in my freezer." **—HBS**

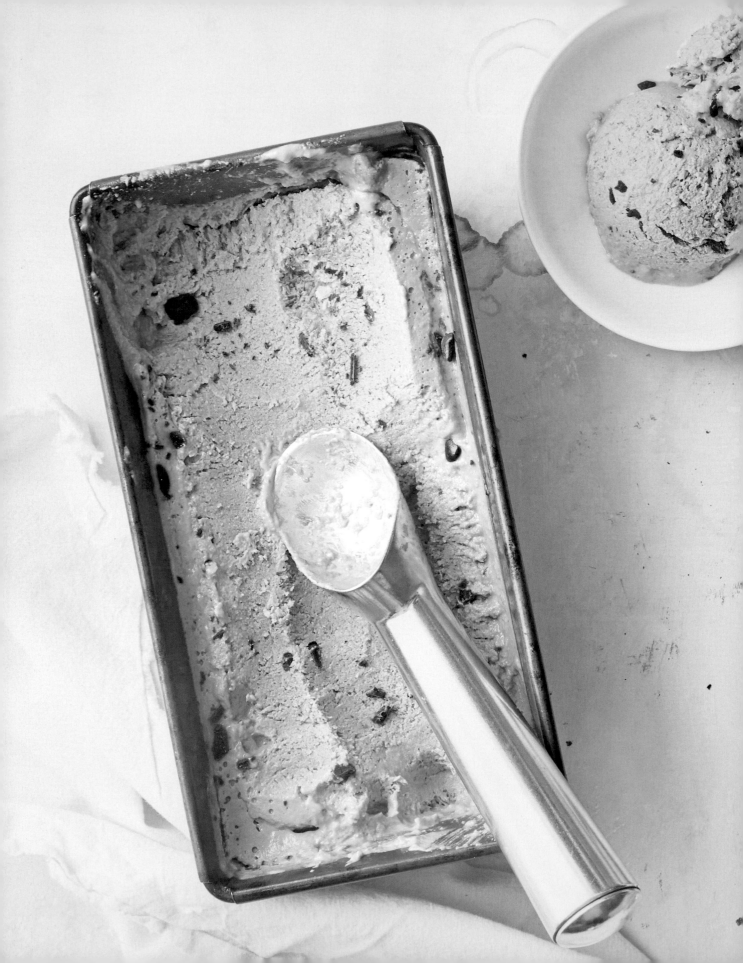

Kale Mint Chocolate Chip Ice Cream

WHEN IT'S A COLD-WEATHER HOLIDAY

It's pretty nuts that the big winter holidays are just a few days out of the year, yet their effects and dominance over our lives go on for months. It doesn't make sense, but it does bring a certain level of cheer, huh? Like the Rockettes at the Macy's Thanksgiving Parade, this well-rehearsed holiday meal provides just the right amount of pizzazz.

All the Fall Feels Salad

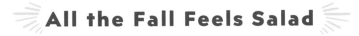

Not all salads are suitable for all seasons. That's where this sweater-season salad comes into play, which is packed with ingredients that your body craves in the fall—the same way we crave fall sweaters. It's been said that it is the perfect marriage of fall flavors. It's also been said that it's impossible to hum while holding your nose. Both of those things are true.

4 LARGE OR 6 TO 8 SMALL SERVINGS

SALAD

1 butternut squash, cut into medium-sized chunks (or a large pre-cut package)

1 15-ounce can of chickpeas, drained and rinsed

1 tablespoon olive oil

½ teaspoon sea salt

½ cup dry quinoa

1 bunch of kale

Fruit—dried cranberries, raisins, apple pieces, and/or pear to taste

Nuts/seeds—raw pumpkin seeds, hemp seeds, sunflower seeds, pecans, and/or walnuts to taste

Goat cheese or dairy-free cheese to taste

MAPLE MUSTARD DRESSING

2 tablespoons Dijon mustard

1 to 2 tablespoons maple syrup

1 tablespoon balsamic vinegar

2 tablespoons olive oil

Pinch of sea salt

1. Preheat the oven to 400°F.
2. In a large bowl, mix the butternut squash, chickpeas, olive oil, and salt.
3. Spread the mixture on a rimmed baking sheet and roast for 20 to 25 minutes, until the squash is tender enough to pierce with a fork and you see some epic charred bits on the edges. You could broil the chickpeas at the end for 3 to 4 minutes to crisp them up a bit.
4. Make the quinoa according to the package instructions.
5. While the quinoa simmers, prep the kale. Tear the leaves off the stems and wash them. Dry the leaves using a salad spinner or a colander and set aside.
6. Make the dressing: Mix the mustard, maple syrup, vinegar, olive oil, and salt together in a jar with a fork, or blend them in a blender.

7. Use your hands to massage 2 tablespoons of the dressing into the kale. Rub the kale for about 2 minutes so it gets soft and turns dark green.

8. Add the cooked quinoa, some squash and chickpeas, a handful or two of seeds/nuts, and a handful or two of fruit. Add more dressing if desired, and eat while wearing a comfy sweater.

HEALTHY EATING ~~**SUCKS**~~**:**

"My guy agrees that even though it's kale, I can bring it to a non-kale kinda crowd at Thanksgiving." **—KH**

"That dressing! I'd eat it on everything!" **—LB**

Massaged Kale Salad

It's possibly depressing that kale gets more massages than you do, but what's not depressing is that you just learned the secret to making kale not suck. Massaging kale with dressing or olive oil and salt (and clean hands) for about two minutes is why, when you eat kale at a restaurant, you like it, but at home, not so much. You know how much your tough muscles love massages? Tough kale does, too. And unlike your muscles that tighten back up like ten minutes later, a massaged kale salad keeps amazingly in your fridge; it won't get soggy like most dressed greens do.

CAUL Me Mashed Potatoes (with Roasted Garlic) or Mashed CauliWOWer

Discovering that cauliflower makes as delectable mashed potatoes as actual potatoes was as mind-blowing as when I found out twins played Michelle Tanner on *Full House*. Much like how my eight-year-old self couldn't spy the difference between Mary-Kate and Ashley, this mashed cauliflower can take the place of mashed potatoes without anyone (your waistline included) being the wiser.

MAKES 4 SERVINGS

ROASTED GARLIC

1 head of garlic

1 tablespoon olive oil

Pinch of pink salt or sea salt

CAULIFLOWER MASH

1 large head of cauliflower, coarsely cut into chunks

¼ cup plain, unsweetened almond milk

3 tablespoons olive oil, plus more to drizzle (optional)

2 teaspoons fresh rosemary or ½ teaspoon dried, plus more as garnish (optional)

2 teaspoon fresh thyme or ½ teaspoon dried, plus more as garnish (optional)

6 to 8 roasted garlic cloves (depending on how much you love garlic)

1½ teaspoons pink salt or sea salt, or to taste

¼ to ½ teaspoon freshly ground black pepper, or to taste

1. Preheat the oven to 400°F.
2. Cut off the end of garlic head to expose the tippy top of the garlic cloves.
3. Place on a big enough piece of aluminum foil to wrap around the whole head.
4. Drizzle the olive oil on top of the garlic and add a pinch of salt.
5. Wrap tightly in the aluminum foil and bake for 40 minutes.
6. When you have about 10 minutes left on the clock, prep the cauliflower mash.
7. Bring a large pot of water to a boil.

8. Add the chunks of cauliflower and cook for 10 minutes or until it's a little soft.

9. Using a slotted spoon, remove the cauliflower to a strainer and let it sit until the roasted garlic is done. Remove the garlic cloves by stabbing them with a fork and sliding them out of the head.

10. Place the cauliflower, almond milk, olive oil, rosemary (if using), thyme (if using), roasted garlic, salt, and pepper in a food processor and process until it's as smooth as mashed potatoes. (You might have to scrape down the sides to make sure every piece of cauli gets in the mix.)

11. Serve as is or add a drizzle of olive oil and an herb sprinkle to up the fancy factor.

LEFTOVERS ARE THE BESTOVERS:

Easily reheat over medium heat for a midday or morning (?) mashed treat.

Save a Turkey, Make Maple Mustard Tempeh

Holiday eating is the epitome of hellthy eating for a lot of us. You hate to reject the main course, but you also hate to sit there getting hangrier by the minute. My solution is to save a turkey and make this tempeh instead! That's right, *and that's how the song goes . . .*

I wish I could take full credit, but this recipe is actually by my plant-food friend mentor (and, serendipitously, my childhood neighbor) Terry Walters, the OG clean eating queen, best-selling author of *Clean Food*, and James Beard Foundation Award finalist for *Clean Start*.

SERVES 4

½ cup olive oil

4 garlic cloves, minced

¼ cup Dijon mustard

¼ cup maple syrup

¼ cup freshly squeezed lime juice

¼ cup tamari

Two 8-ounce packages tempeh

1. Mix the olive oil, garlic, mustard, maple syrup, lime juice, and tamari together in a large bowl.
2. Cut the tempeh into cubes or strips (or turkey shapes?) and add them to the bowl with the marinade.
3. Marinate the tempeh for at least 30 minutes. Preheat the oven to 425°F.
4. Transfer the marinated tempeh to a rimmed baking sheet or a baking dish. Save the remaining marinade. Bake the tempeh for 10 minutes.
5. Flip the tempeh and bake for another 10 minutes.
6. Remove from the oven, transfer to a serving dish, and douse with extra marinade.
7. Refrigerate any leftovers for the bestovers.

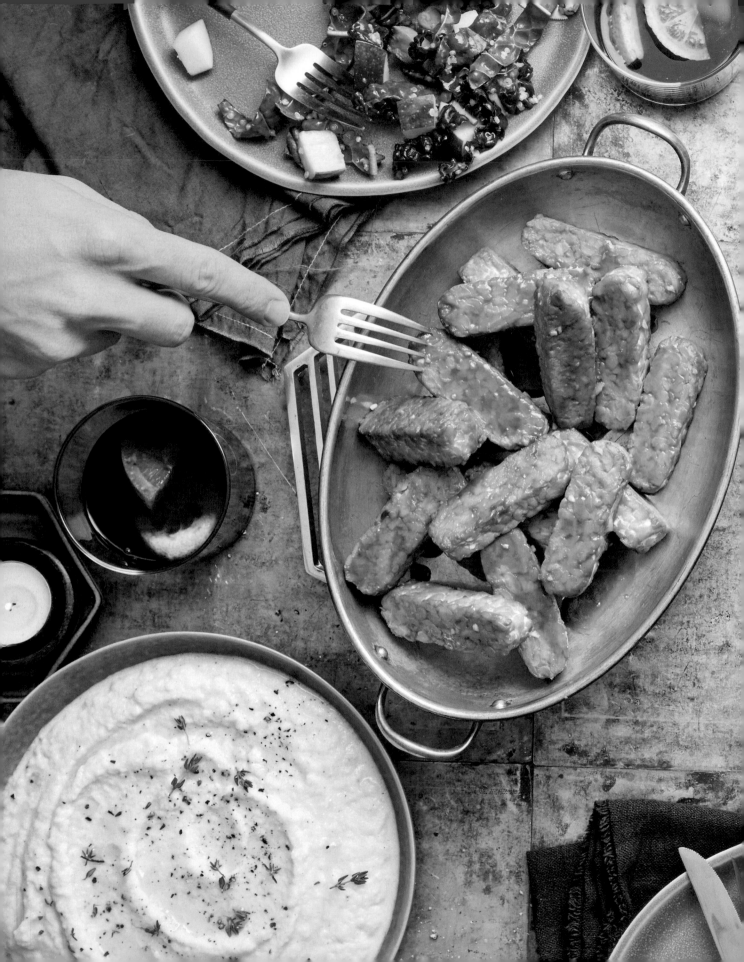

Pictured left to right:
CAUL ME Mashed Potatoes
(with Roasted Garlic) or Mashed
Cauliwower, Save a Turkey,
Make Maple Mustard Tempeh,
All the Fall Feels Salad

No-Family-Drama Mulled Wine

I don't want to jinx it, but ever since I created this recipe, our Thanksgivings have been drama-free. It creates a cozy bubble that no passive-aggressive comments triggering your adolescent wounds can penetrate.

SERVES 8 TO 12

2 bottles red wine, such as Zinfandel

4 cups apple cider

2 to 4 tablespoons agave or maple syrup

Zest and juice of 2 lemons

Zest and juice of 2 oranges

2 cinnamon sticks

4 star anise

10 cloves

8 ounces brandy

Fruit slices, for a garnish

1. In a crockpot (or a pot on the stove), place the wine, cider, agave, lemon juice, and orange juice.
2. Add the lemon zest and orange zest to a cheesecloth.
3. Add the cinnamon sticks, star anise, and cloves to another cheesecloth.
4. Add both to the pot.
5. Cook over low heat (if on the stove) or high (if in a crockpot) for 2 to 4 hours. The liquid shouldn't get feistier than a very low simmer.
6. When you're ready to serve, stir in the brandy and garnish with sliced fruit.

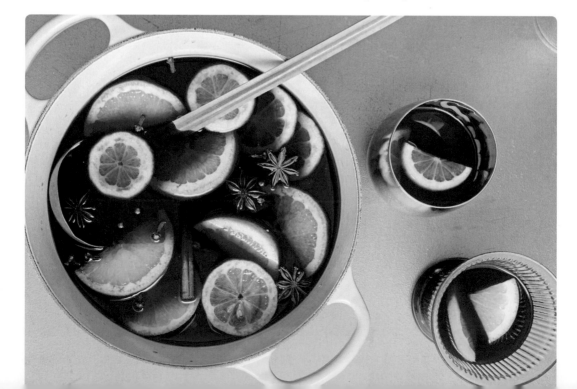

Gooey-gasmic Gingerbread Skillet Cookie

This is one of my favorite recipes. Hands down. Forks up. After photographing it for this book, I slid the leftovers into a ziplock and ate some every night out of the bag like it was dog food. And when I made it for the holidays to enjoy while playing a game called *What Do You Meme?*, my family ate it all before I could finish explaining "meme" to my dad.

SERVES 7 TO 10

1¼ cups packed almond flour (a.k.a. almond meal)

¼ teaspoon baking soda

2 teaspoon ground ginger

1 teaspoon cinnamon

½ teaspoon allspice

½ teaspoon ground cloves

¼ teaspoon nutmeg

½ teaspoon sea salt or pink salt

1 tablespoon flax meal or 1 egg

3 tablespoon melted refined coconut oil, plus more as needed for greasing the pan

⅓ cup maple syrup

⅓ cup molasses

⅓ cup almond butter

1 teaspoon vanilla extract

1 tablespoon almond milk

½ to 1 cup chocolate chips or chunks

1. Lightly oil a pie or tart pan (a round baking pan) with coconut oil spray or coconut oil. Lining it with parchment paper also works.

2. Preheat the oven to 325°F.

3. Mix the almond flour, baking soda, ginger, cinnamon, allspice, cloves, nutmeg, and salt in a large bowl.

4. Make the "flax egg" by mixing the flax meal and 3 tablespoons water together in a small bowl or glass. It's done when the water and flax have turned into a gel. Mix the flax egg, coconut oil, maple syrup, molasses, almond butter, vanilla, and milk in a smaller bowl.

5. Add the wet ingredients to the dry ingredients and combine. Add in the chocolate chips and mix well so they are spread out evenly.

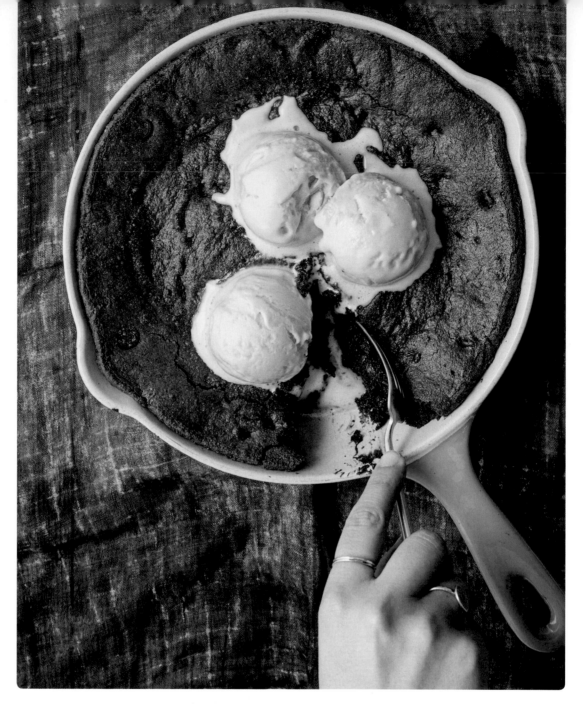

6. Pour the batter into the pie pan and spread it evenly.

7. Bake for 25 minutes. Remove and let cool.

8. Eat with dairy-free vanilla ice cream. (This is optional the way that clothing is
   optional at a clothing-optional hot spring, but then when you wear clothing you're the
   awkward prude non-naked-odd-woman out.)

WHEN IT'S A WARM-WEATHER HOLIDAY, MEANING A POOLSIDE COOKOUT OR PARK BBQ

Even though there are only two true "warm weather holidays," after getting through a gray East Coast winter, any sunny Sunday is a day worth celebrating. So here's a bunch of recipes worth celebrating with. And, really, a bunch of recipes worth celebrating themselves.

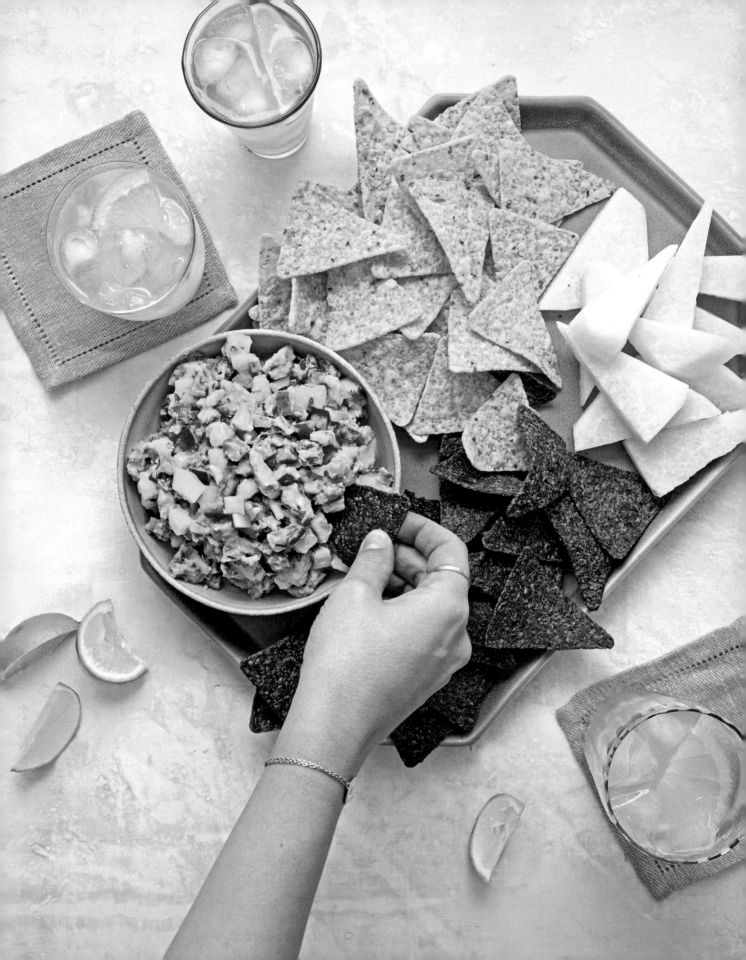

Tropical Guacasalsa

This guacamole-meets-tropical-salsa hybrid is summer in a bite. Or, really, a million bites because it can feed a small army of sun worshippers. It was born out of frustration of trying to dip my chip in salsa and re-dip in guacamole so I could enjoy the natural marriage of the flavors and texture in my mouth. Not only was this an impolite way to muddy the salsa and contaminate the guacamole, but it was a lot of weight for a poor chip to carry. It also was a shampoo and conditioner situation, where, like shampoo, the guac would run out at a much faster rate than the conditioner, i.e., salsa, and then we were left with just salsa. Guacasalsa is delightful on anything summery: veggie burgers, tacos, quesadillas, raw veggies, chips, or just a spoon, and it turns every warm day into a holiday.

SERVES 6 TO 8

2 large or 3 small ripe avocados, flesh scooped out and mashed with a fork

Juice of 2 limes

½ to 1 teaspoon sea salt

1 cup cilantro, chopped (omit if you hate cilantro)

½ cup tomato, chopped

½ cup bell pepper (any color), chopped

½ cup cucumber (peeled if not organic), chopped

½ cup red onion, chopped

1 cup pineapple, chopped

1 cup mango, chopped

1 to 2 jalapeños, with seeds and ribs removed, diced fine (optional)

Combine the avocado, lime juice, cilantro, tomato, bell pepper, cucumber, red onion, pineapple, mango, and jalapeño, if using, in a bowl, mix well, and enjoy on tortilla chips and jicama wedges. Wash down with Coconut Water Margaritas (page 176).

A Lotta Delicious Lemons Walk into This Bar . . .

This recipe has no interesting origin story other than Jesse loves lemon bars, so, honey, this is for you.

16 OR 32 PIECES, DEPENDING ON HOW YOU SLICE 'EM

LEMON LAYER

1½ cups raw cashews

2 tablespoons lemon zest

1½ teaspoons vanilla extract

¼ teaspoon sea salt

⅓ cup maple syrup or honey

⅓ cup freshly squeezed lemon juice
   (from 2 to 3 large lemons)

⅓ cup coconut oil, melted

CRUST

1 cup Medjool dates, pitted

1 cup pecans

½ teaspoon pink salt or sea salt

½ teaspoon vanilla extract

¼ cup shredded unsweetened
   coconut

1 teaspoon lemon zest

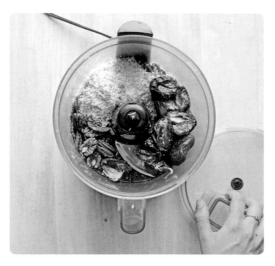
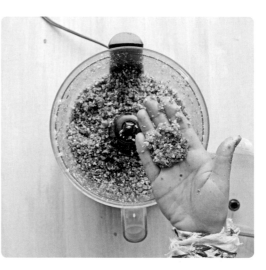

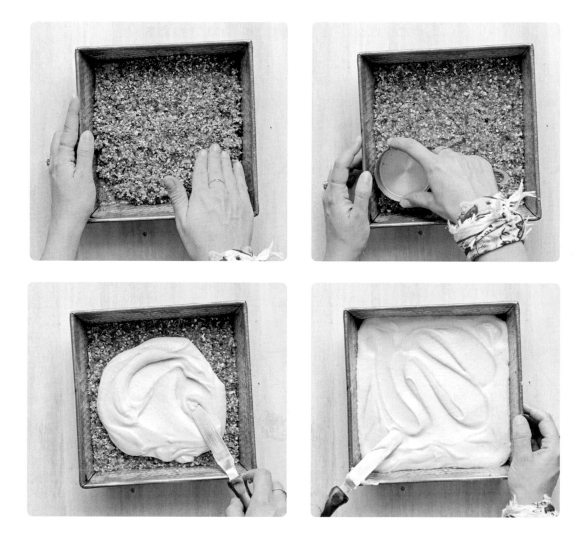

1. Make the lemon layer. Soak the cashews in a bowl of warm water for at least 20 minutes and up to 1 hour.

2. Make the crust: Add the dates, pecans, salt, vanilla, coconut, and lemon zest to a food processor and process well. Press the crust into a 8 x 8-inch dish using the back of a measuring cup. Set aside.

3. Drain and rinse the cashews and place them in a blender. Add the lemon zest, vanilla, salt, maple syrup, lemon juice, and coconut oil. Blend well.

4. Spread this mixture on top of the crust and freeze for 15 to 20 minutes.

5. Remove and let sit on the counter until soft enough to eat or store in the fridge for later. (It'll last about 1 week.)

AFTER [PARTY] THOUGHT:

Vibing with lime? Turn these babies into lime bars by subbing lime zest for the lemon zest and lime juice for lemon juice.

Coconut Water Margarita

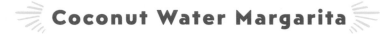

One rainy day in Mexico, Jesse and I took a margarita-making class at our hotel, because he's a tequila aficionado and because I had eyeballed some free guac sitting out for participants. We learned the importance of Cointreau (a brand of orange-flavored liqueur categorized as a triple sec) in a margarita. I also learned that fresh guacamole is a tasty way to distract oneself while one's husband discusses the nuances of different types of tequilas in different types of barrels or whatever. When we came home craving margaritas and wanting to put our multiple bottles of duty-free tequila to good use, we shook up this healthified version using fresh-squeezed orange juice in place of sugar-laden Cointreau, and we've never said hola to another recipe since.

SERVES UNO

Juice of 2 medium limes

Juice of 1 medium orange

4 ounces coconut water

1 shot (⅛ ounce) tequila

Dash of stevia or agave (optional)

1. Stir/mix the lime juice, orange juice, coconut, tequila, and stevia, if using, together in a glass.
2. Add a handful of ice.
3. Stir/mix again.

AFTER [PARTY] THOUGHT:

To serve a pitcher, multiply the above x 4.

AFTER [PARTY] THOUGHT:

Make your batch in the blender, add ice, and you've got a frozen marg.

AFTER [PARTY] THOUGHT:

To make it extra fancy, plop in frozen fruit, muddle some fresh fruit, and garnish with a salted rim or a lime.

Sorry for the three After [party] Thoughts—that margarita went straight to my head.

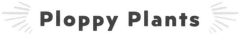

Ploppy Plants

As the urban legend goes, one day a cook named Joe added tomato sauce to a "loose meat sandwich" and born was the "sloppy Joe." Likewise, one day, a person named Talia added tomato sauce and other healthy flavoring agents to lentils and threw in other deliciousness because why not and suddenly, born was Ploppy Plants, which have the same remarkable shirt-staining power as the Joes.

SERVES 5 TO 6

1 cup dry green lentils

1 tablespoon coconut oil or olive oil

2 teaspoons chili powder

2 teaspoons smoked paprika

1 yellow onion, chopped small

4 garlic cloves, minced

1 teaspoon salt, plus a pinch when sautéing the onions and garlic

1 bell pepper (any color), chopped small

1 8-ounce package tempeh

1 huge handful of spinach (about 2 cups), chopped small

1 teaspoon sriracha (or more, if you're a lover!)

1 tablespoon coconut sugar

1 15-ounce can of canned or boxed tomato sauce (not marinara sauce—regular "tomato sauce" in a can, not jar)

Sprouted-grain (like Ezekiel brand) or gluten-free hamburger buns or English muffins (one per person)

Sprouts, as garnish (optional)

Mashed avocados, as garnish (optional)

Sauerkraut, as a garnish (optional)

1. Rinse the lentils in a mesh strainer and then add to a small saucepan with 2 cups of water and bring to a boil. Reduce to a simmer and let the lentils cook, uncovered, until all of the water is absorbed.

2. In a large sauté pan over medium heat, add 1½ teaspoons of the coconut oil, the chili powder, and paprika and sauté the onions and garlic for 3 to 5 minutes, until the onions are translucent. Add a pinch of salt to help expedite this process.

3. Add the bell pepper and continue to sauté.

4. Open the tempeh and use your fingers to crumble the entire package into the pan.

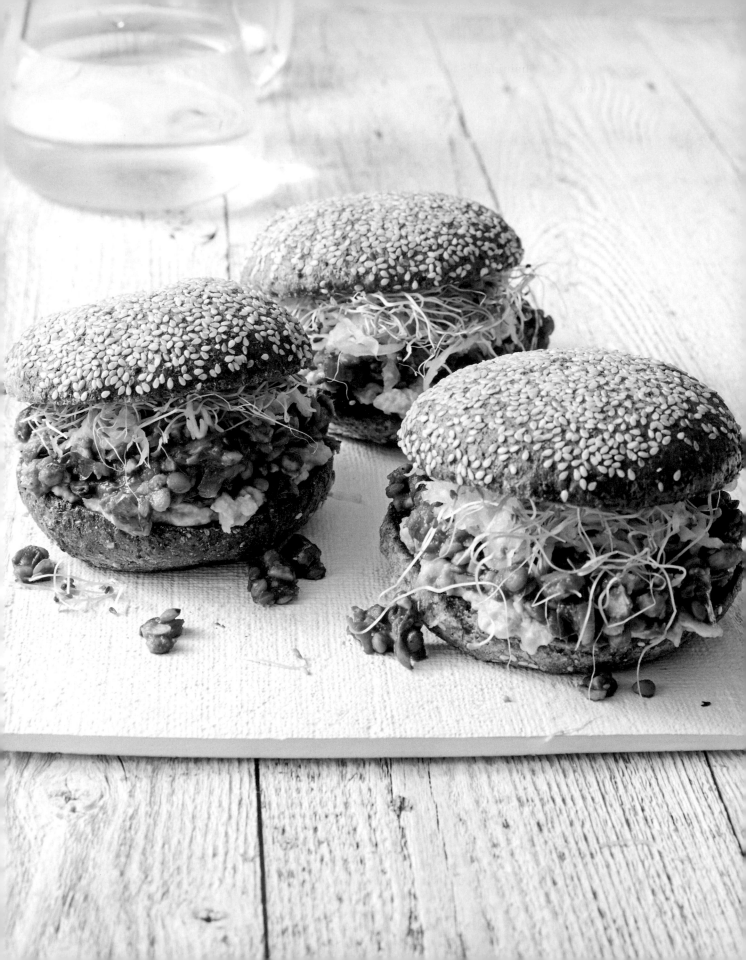

5. Add the remaining 1½ teaspoons coconut oil and sauté over medium-low to medium heat for 5 to 7 minutes.

6. Add the chopped spinach, cooked lentils, salt, sriracha, coconut sugar, and tomato sauce and simmer over low heat for 5 more minutes.

7. Toast the hamburger buns.

8. Remove from the heat and place a heaping portion of those Ploppy Plants onto your buns.

9. Enjoy with sprouts, mashed avocado, and/or sauerkraut.

LEFTOVERS ARE THE BESTOVERS:

Ploppy Plants were *made* for leftovers. If you've got 'em, freeze them or refrigerate them and reheat and enjoy over a bed of greens with sauerkraut and boom! Salad. Or you can heat them up with some zucchini noodles or toss them into a burrito bowl.

AFTER [PARTY] THOUGHT:

Transform into sliders (using small buns) for parties.

HEALTHY EATING ~~SUCKS~~:

"My husband eats like a kid (chicken nuggets and goldfish are a staple) and he loved it!" **—AM**

WHAT TO MAKE WHEN IT'S BRUNCHY, BITCHES

I don't really brunch. Call me jaded or call me someone who doesn't enjoy the need to nap after a midday meal. However, sometimes brunch has to happen and when it does, one or both of these recipes have to get made so this someone will still have energy to be a functioning human after.

'Scuze My French But This French Toast Is F*&king Marvelous!

Growing up, I'd stand on the stepstool to reach the French toast dunking station so I could coat the challah and hand it to my mama for the griddle. But like I outgrew that stepstool, I outgrew eating bread and eggs and milk and butter, and that was a bummer. That's why this banana-based French-ish toast just had to happen.

SERVES 2 TO 3 (MAKES 6 SLICES OF TOAST)

2 cups ripe bananas, peeled and coarsely chopped

⅔ cup plain, unsweetened almond milk

1½ teaspoons cinnamon, plus more to sprinkle

1 teaspoon vanilla extract

6 to 8 ½- to 1-inch slices of day-old bread: whole-grain or gluten-free, just something thick and fluffy. Aim for a thick, fluffy bread—sadly sourdough sours this recipe.

Coconut oil spray, to grease the baking sheet

Maple syrup to taste

Dairy-free yogurt to taste

Your favorite berries

1. Preheat the oven to 350°F.
2. Place the bananas, almond milk, cinnamon, and vanilla in a blender and blend until smooth.
3. Pour the mixture into a bowl large enough and wide enough to fit a slice of bread. A casserole or brownie pan also works brilliantly.
4. Spritz a baking sheet with coconut oil and place the baking sheet nearby and ready to receive your dunked slices of bread.
5. Plop a slice of bread into the batter and count to 10, then flip it and soak the other side for 10 seconds.
6. Gently shake off any excess batter and place the bread slices on the baking sheet. Repeat until you've filled up your entire baking sheet with bread or finished all of your bread.
7. Bake for 15 minutes. Use a spatula to flip the bread and let the other side cook for 10 to 15 minutes, until beautifully golden brown.

NOTE: If you don't have stale bread, bake slices on an ungreased baking sheet at 300°F for 10 to 15 minutes or until the bread starts to feel crusty on both sides.

8. Remove from the oven and serve with maple syrup and/or dairy-free yogurt, a sprinkle of cinnamon, plus a ton of whatever berries and fruit you have and love.

AFTER [PARTY] THOUGHT:

Slice into thin "sticks" for kiddo-friendly French toast fun.

LEFTOVERS ARE THE BESTOVERS:

If you want to add some pizzazz to your weekday brekkies, save some baked Frenchy toast in Tupperware and reheat it in the oven or toaster oven.

HEALTHY EATING ~~SUCKS~~:

"I made it for one of my girlfriends and her boyfriend. Her boyfriend said after his first bite: 'I thought healthy food was supposed to taste like sh*t, but this is actually really good!'" —TZ

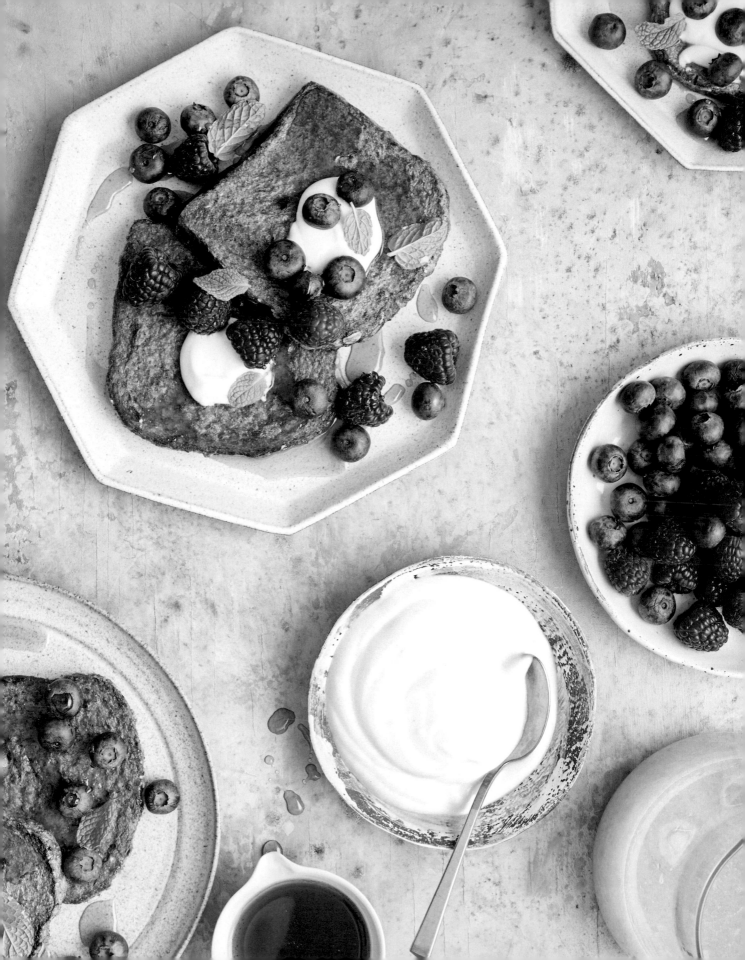

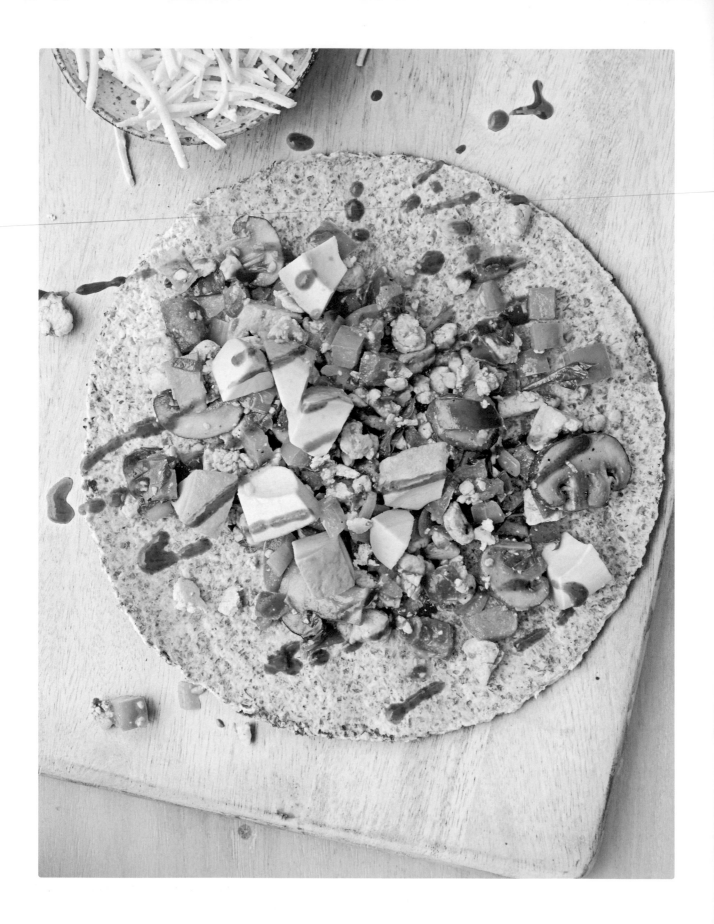

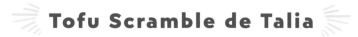

Tofu Scramble de Talia

"The plantier, the merrier" is always my motto, but so is "you do you." Customize away.

MAKES 3 LARGE OR 4 SMALL PORTIONS

Coconut oil spray, for greasing the sauté pan

1 14-ounce package firm or extra-firm tofu

1 medium tomato

1 bell pepper, your favorite color

1 cup mushrooms (optional)

½ yellow or white onion

2 large handfuls of spinach or kale

3 tablespoons nutritional yeast or ½ to 1 cup shredded dairy-free cheese of your choosing

1 teaspoon tamari

½ teaspoon paprika

½ teaspoon garlic powder

Freshly ground black pepper to taste

Sriracha to taste

Avocado, for garnish (optional)

1. Spray a sauté pan with coconut oil. Place the sauté pan on the stove over medium heat.
2. Cut open the package of tofu and drain out the liquid. Place the tofu in the pan and use a spatula to break it into chunks. (The size of your chunks is completely up to you. Freedom! You're welcome.)
3. Cook the tofu while you prep the veggies: Chop the tomatoes, bell pepper, mushrooms, if using, onion, and spinach.
4. Toss the tofu around a bit so it cooks evenly. Add the veggies to the pan. Don't freak out if it seems like a lot of greens; everything will cook down.
5. Add in your flavoring friends: nutritional yeast, tamari, paprika, garlic powder, and black pepper.
6. Mix everything around for 15 minutes.
7. Garnish with Sriracha and avocado, if using.

LEFTOVERS ARE THE BESTOVERS:

If you have leftover scramble (or you want to intentionally make leftover scramble), turn brunch into breakfast by wrapping up Grab and BurritGOs! (page 117) for a ready-to-grab-and-heat weekday delight.

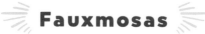

Fauxmosas

Apparently "honeymoon" is slang for "endless free mimosas," which translates to midday blood sugar drops. I've never been a big OJ enthusiast, nor a huge alcohol-before-noon-er, so after our honeymoon, I couldn't even look at the stuff. Ever since, I've been mixing kombucha with grapefruit, my favorite citrus juice (with bonus fat-burning qualities) to give my champagne flutes purpose. (See photo, page 183.)

MAKES 2

⅓ cup ginger kombucha or other kombucha flavor you love, chilled, or chilled Champagne, Cava, or Prosecco

⅓ cup freshly squeezed grapefruit juice or orange juice, chilled

Sprig of thyme to garnish the grapefruit or a slice of orange peel to garnish the orange juice (optional)

1. Combine the kombucha and grapefruit juice in a large glass or small pitcher and mix well (but gently).
2. Pour into two champagne flutes, garnish, and clink 'em!

WHEN IT'S GAME NIGHT— SPORTS ON TV 📺 OR CARDS AGAINST HUMANITY!

There might not be an "I" in team, but there *is* an "I" in win, which is what I *must do*. It's hard not being able to control who touchdowns where, or who chooses my Cards Against Humanity card, but I *can* control what snacks get eaten during games and if it's any from this group, I know it'll count as a victory.

Caramel Fit for a Date

Caramel counting as two or three syllables in charades is the only thing you'll argue about when it comes to this recipe. It's so undeniably fabulous that everyone will be on the same team. Go ahead and roll the dice: For game night this works as a dip for apples or a topping on cheese and crackers, or you can also try it on Apple Nachos (page 87), in Banana Ice Cream (page 110), and mixed into Overnight Oats (page 114).

MAKES A SMALL JAR FULL (ABOUT ¾ CUP)

10 Medjool dates (about 1 cup), pitted

½ teaspoon vanilla extract

1 large pinch sea salt

½ cup plain, unsweetened almond milk

1. Place the dates, vanilla, salt, and almond milk in a blender and blend until creamy.

2. Store in a glass jar in the fridge.

Cauliflower Pizza Poppers

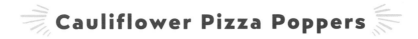

I was going to write about how one of my formative year faves were mini-pizza bagels, and these are even better. But instead, I decided to lead this recipe with this quote from one of my recipe testers, who reported: "These were eaten by three drunk and high twentysomething men and they were so obsessed with them LOL."—AC.

Sold.

SERVES 4

2 heads of cauliflower

1 tablespoon olive oil

1 14-ounce jar pizza sauce

1½ cups raw cashews

¼ cup nutritional yeast

½ teaspoon pink salt or sea salt

½ to 1 cup fresh basil, or to taste

1. Preheat the oven to 425°F.
2. Wash the cauliflower and remove the green leafy part. Chop into medium-large florets and place in a large bowl. Drizzle with the olive oil and the pizza sauce and toss well so that each floret is generously coated with sauce. #nofloretleftbehind
3. In a food processor, process the cashews, nutritional yeast, and salt until it's a coarse, sandy texture. Set aside.
4. Place the florets on two rimmed baking sheets. (One baking sheet is perfect for 1 head of cauliflower.)
5. Use a spoon to spread a generous amount of the cashew cheese crumbles on top of the cauliflower, using the pizza sauce to serve as the "glue" to help them stick.
6. Bake for 30 to 35 minutes. They're done when a fork pokes through a floret easily and they're starting to crisp on the bottom.
7. While the cauliflower is baking, rinse, dry, and chop the basil as small as you can.
8. Remove the cauliflower from the oven, sprinkle fresh basil on top, and then ready, set, serve.
9. Store leftovers in a closed container in the fridge.

AFTER [PARTY] THOUGHT:

If you're into spice, give these guys a kick by sprinkling them with red pepper flakes.

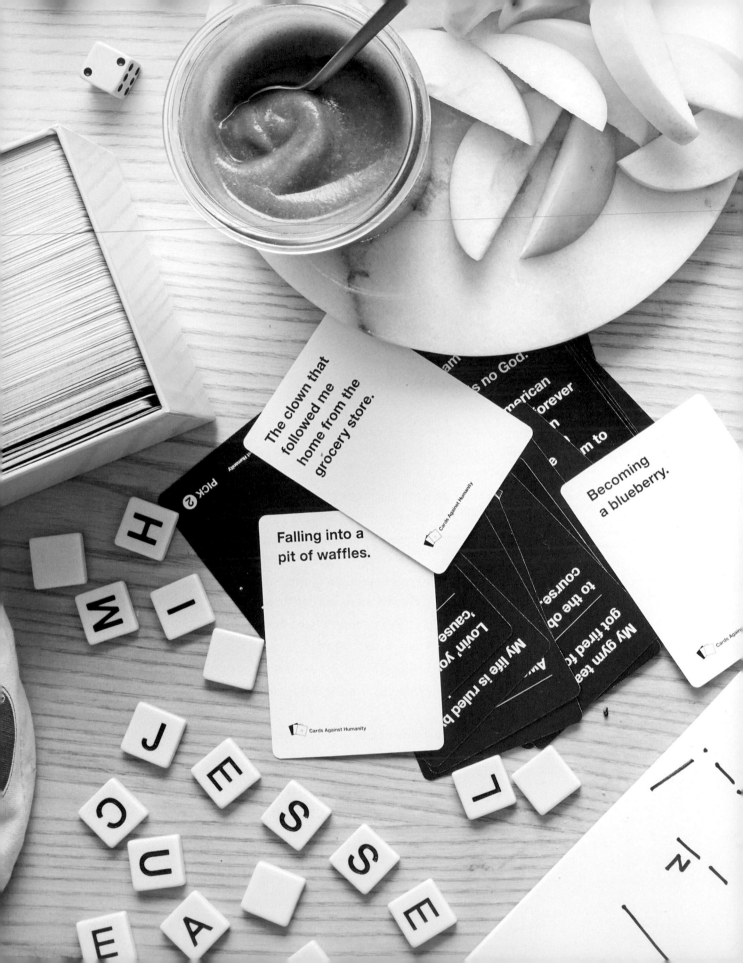

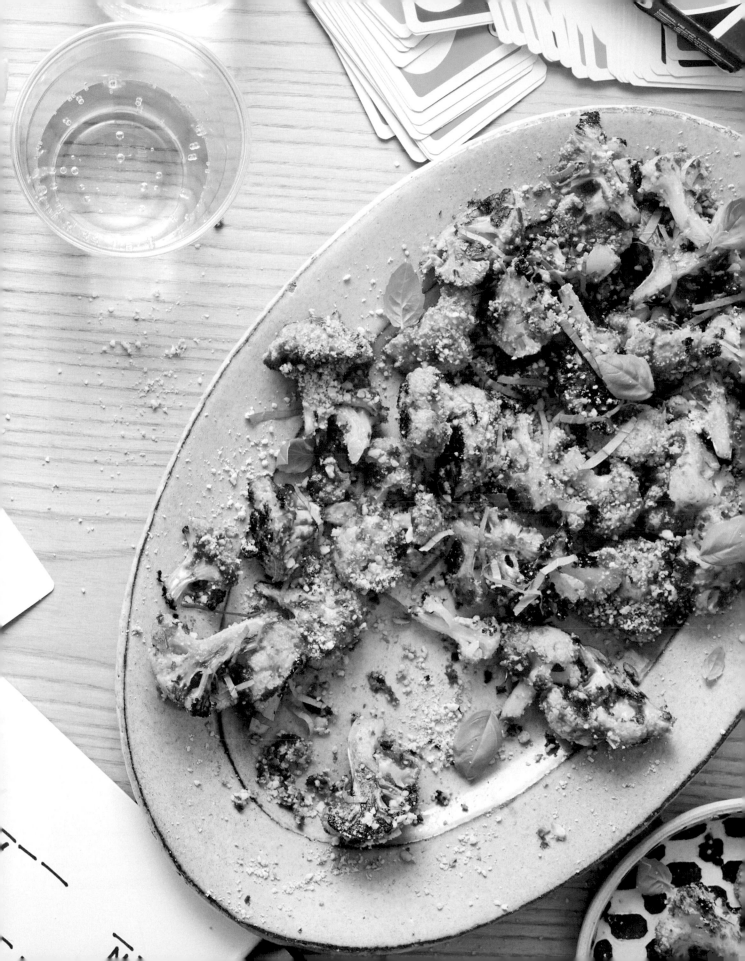

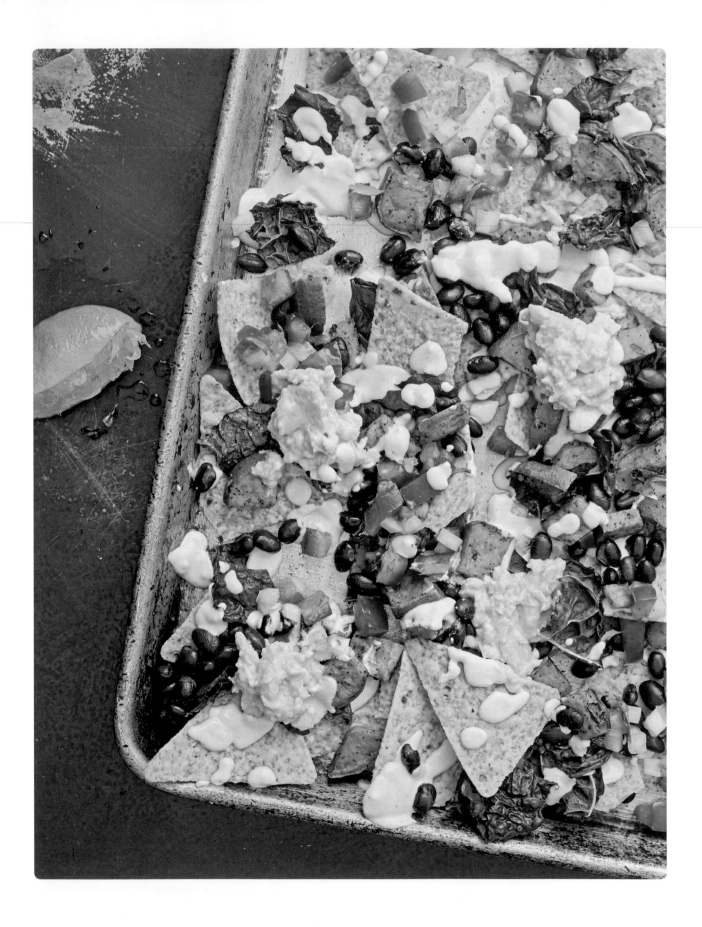

Nacho-Unhealthy Nachos

In sports, a hat trick means three feats in one game, like a soccer player scoring three goals or a hockey player scoring . . . three goals. In nachos, a hat trick means three feats in one recipe, like how this is crap-free, flavor-full, *and* plant-packed.

SERVES A BUNCH OF BITES FOR A BUNCH OF PEOPLE

2 medium sweet potatoes or 3 cups butternut squash, chopped into small cubes

4½ teaspoons extra-virgin olive oil

½ teaspoon ground chili powder

2 pinches of salt

3 to 4 cups dino kale, cut into small slices

1 bag of your favorite tortilla chips

1 batch of Liquid Gold Cheese Sauce (page 55)

1 15-ounce can black beans or pinto beans, drained and rinsed

Guac-ish (see page 193)

1 16-ounce jar of your favorite salsa or pico de gallo

1. Preheat the oven to 400°F.

2. In a large bowl, toss the sweet potato cubes with 1 tablespoon of the olive oil, then add the chili powder and salt and toss some more.

3. Spread the sweet potatoes on a rimmed baking sheet and roast for about 25 minutes, until golden and tender. At the 15-minute mark, flip the baking sheet around so the sweet potatoes cook evenly. Add the kale.

4. After 10 more minutes, remove the baking sheet from the oven and set aside. Reduce the oven temperature to 350°F.

5. On a baking sheet lined with parchment paper, spread out the bag of tortilla chips. Drizzle with the cheese sauce. Add the sweet potato chunks and kale, followed by the beans, and then another cheese drizzle.

6. Pop into your oven for 8 minutes.

7. Eight minutes is plenty of time for you to make Guac-ish. Do that!

8. Remove the nachos from the oven, dollop the guac all over, followed by the salsa, and then dive in.

9. Leftover cheese can be saved in a sealed jar in the fridge for about 5 days.

LEFTOVERS ARE THE BESTOVERS:

Save any leftovers in a sealed container in the fridge.
Trust me on this. And yes, I eat them cold.

WHAT TO MAKE WHEN SOMETHING GIRLY'S GOING ON

I'm not the girliest of girls. I skipped having a bridal shower, dropped out of my college sorority after a month (but still wear the incredibly comfy Alpha Phi T-shirts around my home), and have never once thrown a "girl's night," but if doing so is an excuse to eat these pink treats, then let me fluff my pillows and cue up *The Notebook*.

Strawberry Hummus with Homemade Cinnamon Sugar Chips

1 cup canned chickpeas, drained and rinsed

1 cup chopped strawberries

2 tablespoons maple syrup

¼ cup almond butter

Pinch of sea salt

1 teaspoon vanilla extract

1 to 2 tablespoons almond milk (optional)

½ teaspoon strawberry extract (optional)

Chopped strawberries, for garnish

continued

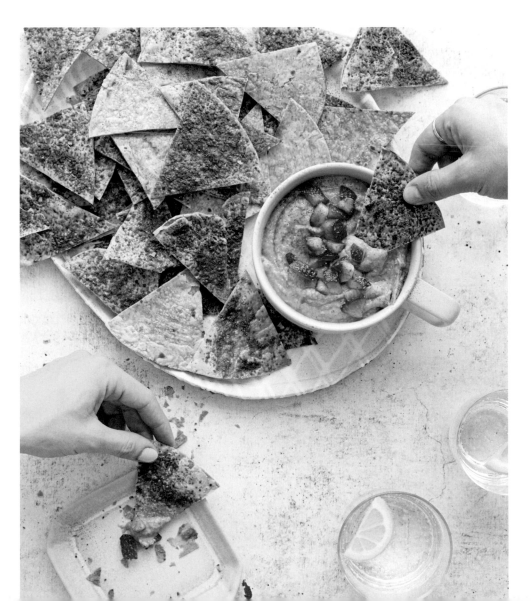

1. Process the chickpeas, strawberries, maple syrup, almond butter, salt, vanilla, almond milk, if using, and strawberry extract, if desired in a food processor until well combined. Add almond milk if it's too thick.

2. Transfer to a jar or bowl and garnish with chopped strawberries. Store leftovers covered in the fridge for up to 5 days.

CINNAMON SUGAR CHIPS

6 spelt or sprouted-grain tortillas

1 teaspoon cinnamon

3 tablespoons coconut sugar

Coconut oil spray

1. Preheat the oven to 350°F. Spray a baking sheet with coconut oil spray.

2. Slice the tortillas into triangles—or use a heart-shaped cookie cutter.

3. Mix together the cinnamon and coconut sugar in a small bowl.

4. Lay down all your chips on the baking sheet.

5. Spray the top of the chips with coconut oil, then sprinkle on the cinnamon sugar topping.

6. Bake for 8 to 16 minutes. Stand by so they get crispy but don't burn—the baking time will vary based on the tortillas and the oven. You want the tortillas lightly golden brown.

HEALTHY EATING ~~SUCKS~~:

"I made it for my partner, whose favorite meal is steak and potatoes and who definitely doesn't like beans, and wow. She went back for seconds and thirds because she genuinely loved it! This was a definite win." —ML

LEFTOVERS ARE THE BESTOVERS:

This hummus tastes even better after sitting in the fridge overnight and is 100 percent better than PB&J on toast.

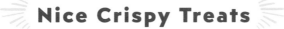

Nice Crispy Treats

Even as a tot who had no clue about the inner ecosystem of my body, I knew that a sticky marshmallowy chunk in a blue shiny label, which I'd sometimes lick off the label like the savage summer day camper I was, made me feel gross. But nothing could beat that crispy texture bound together by a should-be-illegal amount of sugar so I kept plowing Rice Krispies Treats down. Now, I can't even look at those blue shiny labels without feeling nauseous, but still nothing beats that texture and taste—except these.

SERVES 9, 16, OR 20, DEPENDING ON HOW SMALL (OR LARGE) YOU CUT THE TREATS

½ cup nut or seed butter (chunky or smooth)

½ cup brown rice syrup, honey, coconut nectar, or maple syrup

1 tablespoon coconut oil

1 teaspoon vanilla extract

2 pinches of sea salt

3 cups brown rice krispies (not puffed rice cereal)

Chocolate chips, colorful sprinkles, or coconut flakes (optional)

continued

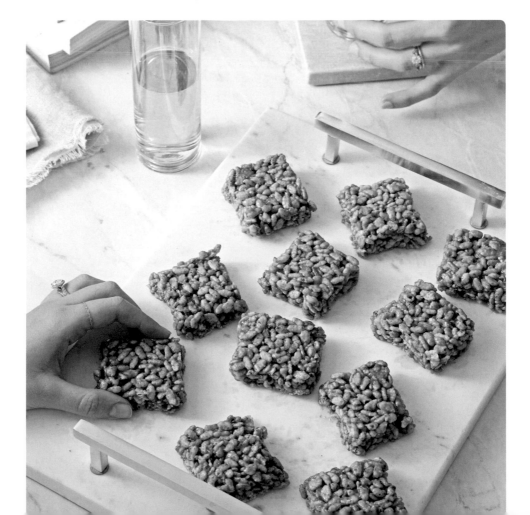

1. Line an 8 x 8-inch or 9 x 9-inch pan with parchment paper.

2. In a medium pot on the stove over low heat, place the nut butter, brown rice syrup, coconut oil, vanilla, and salt. Or combine the ingredients in a microwave-safe dish and zap them in the microwave until melted.

3. Stir until all of the ingredients have melted together. Let them cool for a sec (not too long or they'll get too sticky).

4. Stir in the krispies, and, if you want, add in a bonus treat. Press the coated krispies into the prepared pan and slide it into the freezer for about 10 minutes. Then remove, slice into squares, and serve.

AFTER [PARTY] THOUGHT:

This is an order: Do not limit these to girly happenings; they're
a divine snack for family movie night, a party, a work potluck, kiddos'
soccer games, babysitting, and outdoor adventures like camping.

WHEN YOU'RE GOING TO A POTLUCK WITH FOLKS YOU DON'T KNOW THAT WELL

Even though I'm plenty proud of my plant-eating ways, sometimes I don't want to be loud about it. I don't want it to be the topic of conversation, or someone's first impression. I imagine it's similar to an adult movie actress who doesn't necessarily want her line of work to be the topic of her neighborhood potluck, so she wears a shlubby sweater and lays low. You can just slide any of these dishes onto the table, low key, without being called out as The Healthy Eater—but on which you know you can safely go back for thirds.

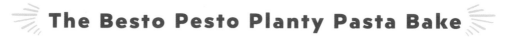

The Besto Pesto Planty Pasta Bake

SERVES 3 OR 4 AS A SIDE

½ cup raw walnuts

1 8-ounce box of pasta (I love a high-protein variety like Banza Chickpea Pasta)

3 cups spinach

1 cup basil, tightly packed

2 garlic cloves

Juice of ½ to 1 lemon

¼ teaspoon sea salt or pink salt

¼ cup olive oil

2 tablespoons nutritional yeast or pecorino cheese, plus more for topping

2 cups frozen broccoli

1 cup frozen peas

1 cup sun-dried tomatoes, chopped

1. Preheat the oven to 400°F.
2. Bring a large pot of water to a boil.
3. Spread the walnuts on an ungreased baking sheet and toast for 5 to 8 minutes, until they smell amazing and are lightly brown. Let 'em cool.
4. When the water boils, add the pasta and cook according to the package directions. Drain and rinse the pasta and return it to the pot.
5. Place the spinach, walnuts, basil, garlic, lemon juice, salt, olive oil, and nutritional yeast in a food processor and process them until creamy, pausing to scrape down the sides as needed.
6. Add the frozen broccoli and peas to a small pot. Add enough water to cover and bring to a boil, then drain.
7. Toss the cooked pasta with the pesto, and add in the peas, broccoli, and sun-dried tomatoes. Add 3 or 4 tablespoons of water, 1 tablespoon at a time, to make it a little saucy. Stir well to combine.
8. Transfer this plant party to a casserole or baking dish and sprinkle with more nutritional yeast—as much as you want.
9. Bake for 10 minutes and remove and serve immediately.
10. Store leftovers in a covered container in your fridge.

HEALTHY EATING ~~SUCKS~~:

"I dipped my finger into the pesto before mixing it into the pasta and almost fell over, it tasted so good." **—TZ**

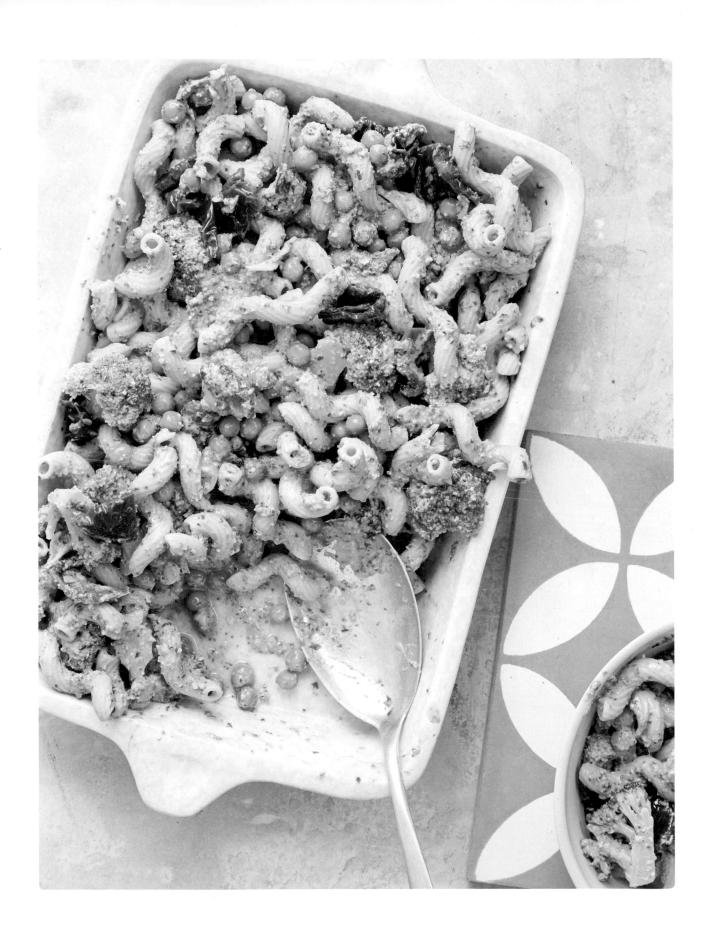

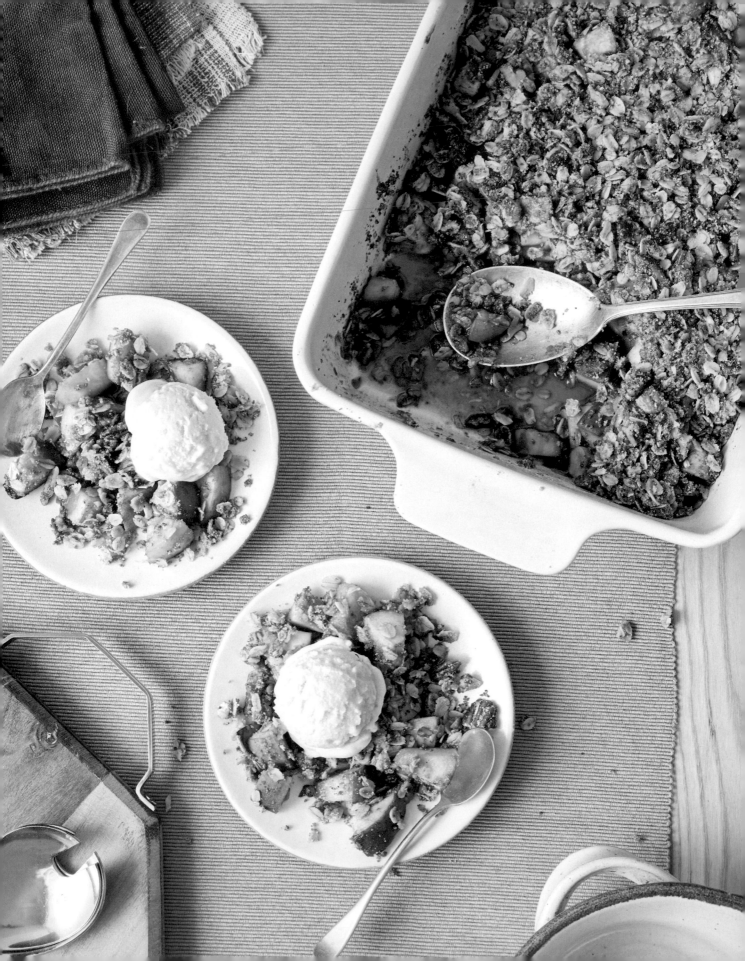

BERRY Good, PEACHy Perfect, or Beyond APPLE-ing Crisp

Part of the fun of this recipe is the fruity flexibility it allows for. Go buck wild mixing and matching whatever is in season.

SERVES ABOUT 6

Coconut oil spray, to grease the pan

5 cups berries, chopped peaches, or chopped apples

2 tablespoons plus ⅓ cup coconut sugar

1 cup rolled oats

½ cup almond flour (a.k.a. almond meal)

½ cup chopped pecans

¼ teaspoon sea salt

1½ teaspoons cinnamon (optional)

1 teaspoon ground ginger (optional)

¼ cup coconut oil (at room temperature—solid, not melted)

2 to 3 tablespoons unsweetened coconut flakes (optional)

Dairy-free ice cream or Cashew Sweet Cream (recipe below) for serving

1. Preheat the oven to 350°F.
2. Grab a baking dish and spray or smother it with coconut oil.
3. Add the chopped fruit and spread it out.
4. Drizzle 2 tablespoons of the coconut sugar on top.
5. In a large bowl, mix together the oats, almond flour, pecans, the remaining ⅓ cup coconut sugar, and the salt. Add the cinnamon, ginger, and coconut flakes, if using.
6. Use your clean hands to massage the coconut oil into the mixture.
7. Place on top of the fruit and spread evenly.
8. Bake for 40 to 50 minutes, until the crisp topping is golden.
9. Portion out and top with dairy-free ice cream or cashew cream.

CASHEW SWEET CREAM:

1 cup raw cashews

2 to 4 tablespoons maple syrup or to taste

1 teaspoon vanilla extract

¼ teaspoon sea salt

continued

1. Soak the cashews in warm/room-temperature water in a bowl for at least 2 hours to overnight. Drain and rinse.

2. Blend the cashews, ½ cup water, maple syrup, vanilla, and salt in a blender for about 2 minutes. Add more water, a tablespoon at a time, if you want a thinner cream.

3. Transfer to the fridge to chill until desired temperature (the freezer's cool, too—*pun intended*—if you need to chill the cream quickly).

4. Dollop and serve.

How to Not Spend Your 401(k) on Food

Last summer, I was doing one of my weekly group coaching sessions. At the start of each video call, I'd ask people to share a win from the week since our last chat. I was always blown away. Six pounds lost. Energy skyrocketing. Quality of sleep was like . . . day and night . . . with an easy good night. Here's the thing: I hadn't introduced them to some MCT oil superfood Venezuelan concoction or fancy pants expensive fairy dust.

This is the real secret when it comes to "wellness": Good health don't cost a thing. *(Sung in your head—or out loud—to JLo's 2001 hit "Love Don't Cost a Thing.")* It's not the well-marketed or cleverly branded or nifty packaged things that bring you true wellness. The wellness industry is exactly that—an industry. That makes money. Billions of dollars of it. Thanks to you and me.

Have you heard of nutrient density? It's the number of nutrients you get per calorie. It doesn't have anything to do with macronutrients (proteins, fat, carbs). It's about micro-nutrients: vitamins, minerals, antioxidants, and phytochemicals. These are essential for our bodies to thrive. Nutrient-dense foods give us the most nutrition for our literal buck. If you have money burning a hole in your pocket, spend it on organic sweet potatoes instead of conventional ones, or quinoa instead of white rice, or kombucha instead of Fanta. We're talking the difference of a dollar or two.

There are also a lot of what I'd call pseudo-plants out there. I'm talking about the bars, the powders, the bottles. I'm glad that some corporations have woken to the fact that a lot of us would prefer higher-quality processed food—but it's still processed food. It's cool to eat this stuff once in a while—I certainly do—but try not to fool yourself into thinking that you're beating the system. Cupcakes, even gluten-free carrot ones, are not as nutritious as an actual carrot, okay? Don't panic; just be mindful.

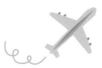

WHEN YOUR BANK ACCOUNT IS VERTICALLY CHALLENGED

When money is tight, or time is, I rely on toast to get me through. Think outside the bread box. Use sourdough, sprouted-grain, or gluten-free bread; a sprouted-grain or brown rice tortilla; or even a rice cake. Here are twenty toast ideas for penny-pinching plant parties on your plate:

Toast Twenty Ways

1. Peanut butter + cilantro + a drizzle of sriracha

2. Nut butter + mashed raspberries, blackberries, or blueberries + a sprinkle of chia seeds

3. Nut butter + sliced banana toast + a sprinkle of cinnamon (and maybe a couple of chocolate chips or cacao nibs)

4. Tahini + sliced apple toast + a drizzle of honey

5. Mashed avocado + black beans or refried beans + sprouts + hot sauce

6. Avocado (mashed with a fork) + a sprinkle of sea salt + a sprinkle of red pepper flakes

7. Hummus + cucumber + hemp seeds

8. Avocado + leftover TGIT tempeh (page 47) + sauerkraut

9. Tahini Miso Magic Sauce (page 273) + shredded carrots + edamame

10. Pumpkin

11. Peanut butter + chocolate chips

12. Pesto + chopped veggie burger + hemp seeds

13. Tahini Miso Magic Sauce (page 273) + leftover Camo Tofu (page 48)

14. Coconut yogurt or goat cheese + sautéed mushrooms + sea salt + parsley + olive oil

15. Pumpkin puree + cinnamon + nutmeg + cloves + pinch of sea salt + drizzle of maple syrup

16. Dairy-free yogurt + sliced strawberries + sprinkle of chia seeds

17. Dairy-free cream cheese or goat cheese + sliced tomatoes + chopped basil + black pepper + sea salt

18. Pesto (page 200) + roasted chickpeas (roasted at 425°F for 15 minutes) + sea salt

19. Leftover mashed sweet potato + black beans + avocado + chili powder

20. Leftover mashed sweet potato + tahini drizzle + nutritional yeast + roasted chickpeas (roasted at 425°F for 15 minutes)

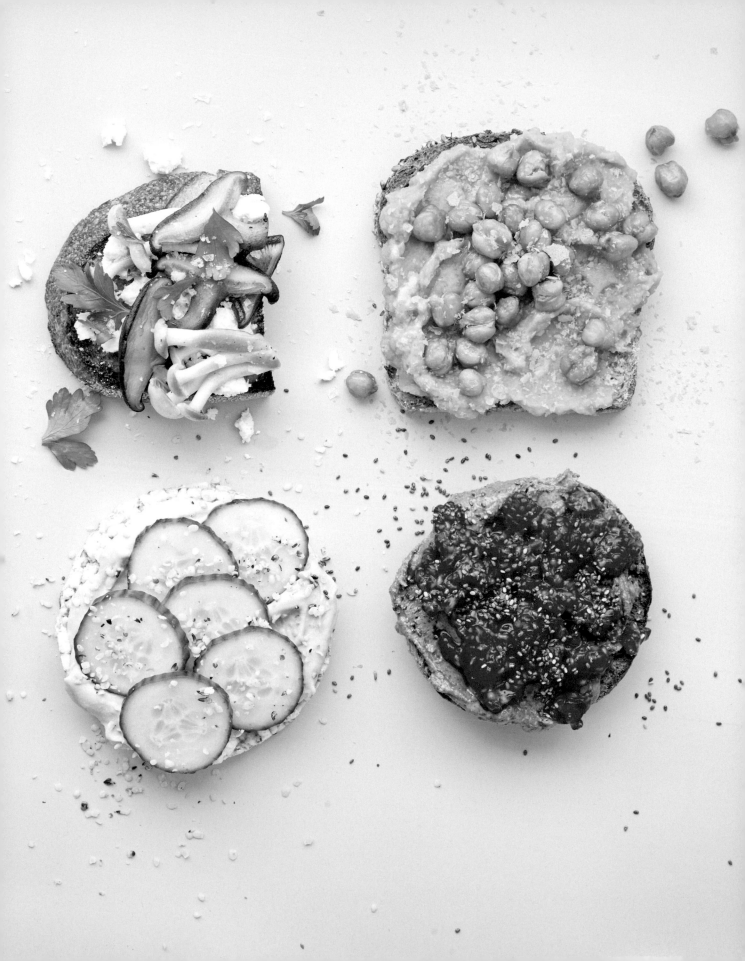

YOU JUST WANT TO MAKE PLAIN PLANTS TASTE GREAT

Even though, yes, absolutely, we're all beautiful and worthy and perfectly imperfect just the way we are, we can all benefit from a little liquid concealer sometimes. Same with plants. Perfect pure, yes, but sometimes better with some sauces? Also yes. Here are my favorite quick tricks to gussy up on plain plants and to use in bowlin' (page 99).

Red Peppa Pesto

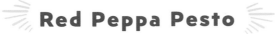

This unique pesto is the Enya of flavors, able to harmonize with any meal. Use it to:

Drizzle on roasted veggies. Mix into pasta with peas and tempeh (page 47).

Spread onto a wrap (like hummus) with beans and veggies. Toss over spaghetti squash with white beans, sautéed mushrooms, and onions with spinach.

Use as a topping for eggs. Smear on burgers and avocado toast. Dollop on grilled veggies. Spread on pitas with spinach, a veggie burger, and pickles. Use as a dip with veggies, crackers, and crudité. Put on zoodles with tomatoes and kale and Camo Tofu (page 48). Mixed into quinoa. As a dip with chips or Eggplant Fries (page 138).

MAKES ABOUT 2½ CUPS OR ABOUT A 10½-OUNCE JAR FULL

½ cup raw almonds

1 cup roasted red peppers (in a 10½-ounce jar packed with water or olive oil)

2 tablespoons nutritional yeast, optional

½ teaspoon sea or pink salt

¼ teaspoon freshly ground black pepper

¼ to ½ teaspoons red pepper flakes or smoked paprika (optional)

2 to 4 tablespoons water

1. Preheat the oven to 325°F. Spread the almonds out on a baking sheet. Bake for 5 minutes or until you can smell them all toasty and delicious.

2. Remove the roasted red peppers from the jar with a fork. You don't want to use the extra oil in the jar (save it for a salad mixed with balsamic vinegar later).

3. Add the almonds, peppers, nutritional yeast, if using, salt, pepper, and red pepper flakes, if using, to a blender and blend. Add water in tablespoon increments until you get your desired texture.

4. Now, what plants to serve it on? That's up to you.

HEALTHY EATING SUCKS:

"My husband doesn't love pesto, but I'm trying to turn him on to it. However, this was a huge hit. This entire thing was literally gone within the day. I'll have to triple the recipe next time. I will make this every week for the rest of my life, it was that good." —**EP**

LEFTOVERS ARE THE BESTOVERS:

Keep leftovers in a sealed container in your fridge (maybe even in the now-empty red pepper jar). Use this sauce in any of the aforementioned suggested ways, or come up with your own N-Z ideas.

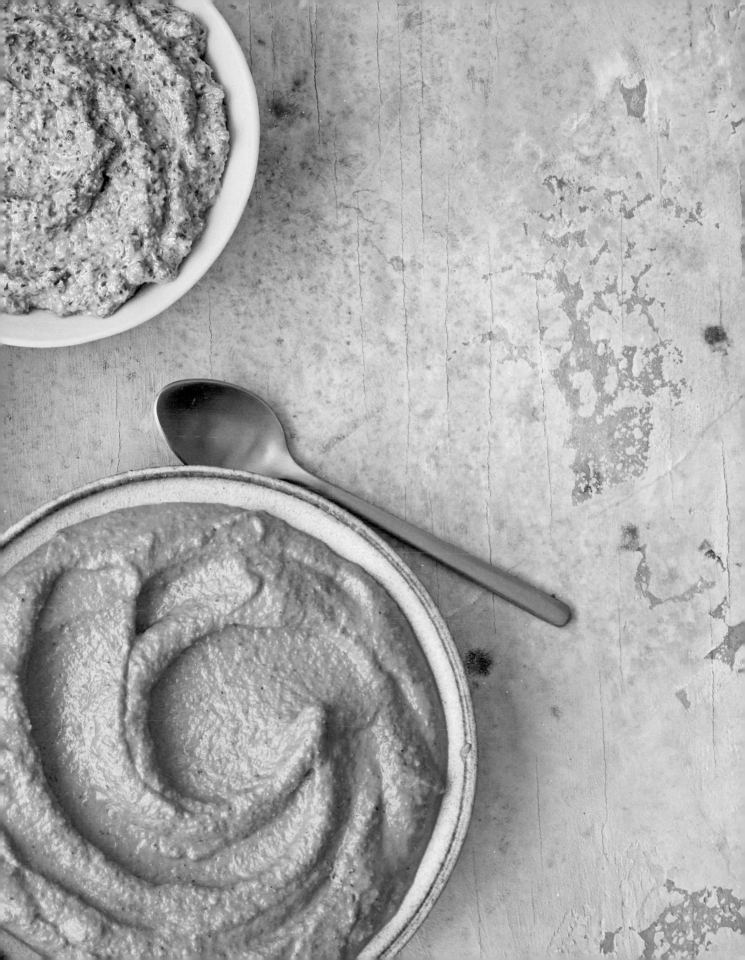

My Besto Planty Pesto Formula

I'd still be trying to pass high school physics if I hadn't snuck formulas in my graphic calculator (sorry, Mr. Zlatin!), but this is one equation I have down pat. It results in a sauce you can use to heighten any roasted plant, sandwich, wrap, pasta, pizza, or bland bowl of quinoa or rice. Beat that, relative velocity.

Step 1: Choose herb: 3 cups of basil, parsley, cilantro, or combo.

Step 2: Add fat: ½ ripe avocado or ½ cup of raw or lightly toasted cashews, pine nuts, walnuts or pumpkin seeds.

Step 3: Get it wet: 3 to 4 tablespoons of olive oil.

Step 4: Add a kick: 1 to 2 peeled garlic cloves and the juice of ½ to 1 whole lemon.

Step 5: Add spice: salt and freshly ground black pepper to taste plus 2 to 4 tablespoons nutritional yeast or pecorino cheese.

Step 6: Sneak in the super stuff: 2 to 3 cups washed and dried kale or spinach.

Pick your plants à la the equation above.

Throw them in your food processor and process, pausing to scrape down the sides as needed. Add to the food you're making so it'll taste amazing and store leftovers in a sealed jar in the fridge for 5 days.

Your Greens' New Go-To DRESSing

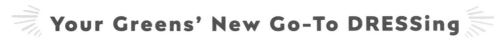

Meet my little black dress[ing]. This sexy number comes together easily and fits almost every occasion, and just like that dress matches every heel and purse, it has yet to find a meal it doesn't liven up.

MAKES ABOUT 1 CUP

½ cup mashed ripe avocado (a little less than 1 whole avocado)

2 to 3 garlic cloves, chopped

2 tablespoon apple cider vinegar

1 tablespoon tahini

1 teaspoon Dijon mustard

2 tablespoons nutritional yeast

½ teaspoon sea salt or pink salt

Water (added one splash at a time if you like a thinner dressing)

1. Combine the avocado, garlic, apple cider vinegar, tahini, mustard, nutritional yeast, salt, and water in a high-speed blender and blend until smooth.

2. Store leftover dressing sealed in the fridge for up to 1 week.

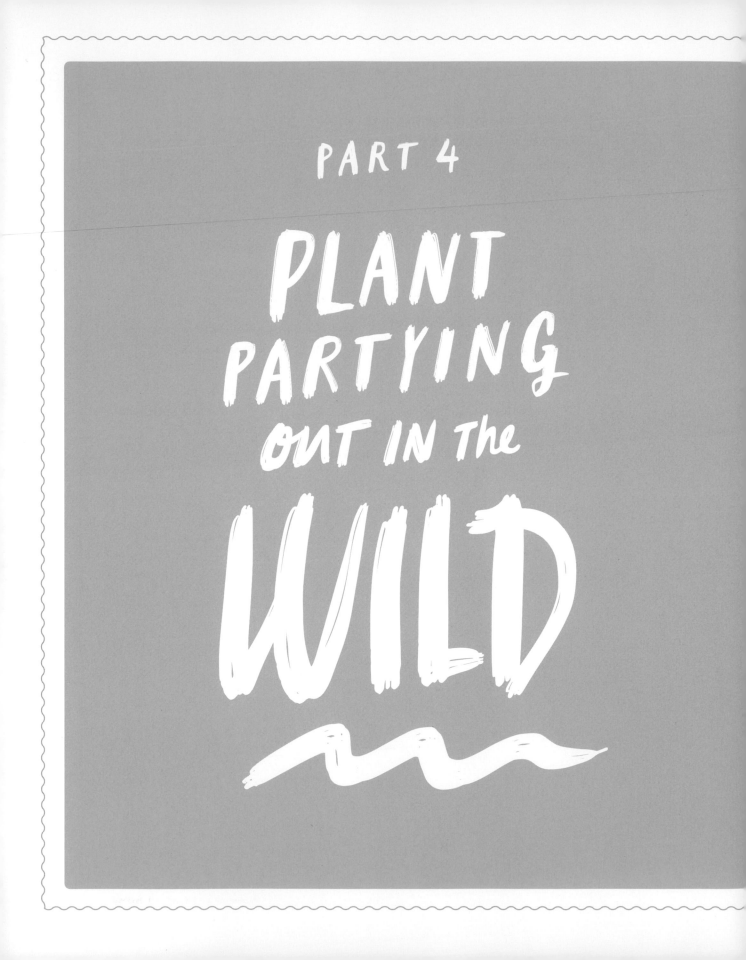

PART 4

PLANT PARTYING OUT IN THE WILD

(in the "eating is an activity" social circus that is our world)

Food is personal and private. It's also social and public. It's weird like that. My hope is that, as you venture out into the world eating the way that makes you and your body happy, you feel empowered to stay in your own lane, stay on your own yoga mat, focus on your own fork. As Theodore Roosevelt once said: "Comparison is the thief of joy." And as I've been known to add: "It's also stupid."

If someone gives you crap via words or looks, I am telling you, based on years of first-hand experience, it's because they feel like crap themselves and have a crap-ton of guilt and jealousy that you're successfully doing what they instinctively know they should try. So just do you.

How to Eat at a Restaurant When It Looks Like There's Zero on the Menu for You

Maybe as soon as you peep the menu and don't spot "quinoa" or "kale," you either give up and eat a cheeseburger and onion rings or play it safe and order the most boring house salad ever. Which you season with your tears.

When we find ourselves without obvious options, it's up to us to work a little magic so we don't end up getting a "house salad with oil and vinegar, hold the cheese, please." Here's my step-by-step strategy for putting together a delicious meal no matter what booth your butt is in:

STEP 1: Scan the salads. The first place your eyes should go is to the salads. See if the restaurant can offer you one hearty enough to be a meal, or if they only have salads that can suffice as a side. This will dictate the rest of your menu search. If you find a salad that's offered as an app and that's chock-full of veggies and clean proteins like black beans, a veggie burger, chickpeas, or salmon if you eat fish, go ahead right and order (with a non-creamy dressing, and add avocado to bulk it up, too).

STEP 2: Browse the burgers. If the restaurant serves burgers, this is your next stop. If they have a veggie burger, congrats, you've won the plant-party lottery. Confirm with your server that it's not made with anything you're avoiding (cheese, egg, soy, seitan—a.k.a. gluten), ask for a salad or veggies as a side instead of fries, and you're good to go.

Even better, avoid the bun and get the veggie burger *on* a salad.

STEP 3: See the sides. Sides are generally where all the vegetables are, and it's easy and satisfying to order a whole bunch as your meal. Many places offer at least one side of greens, like spinach or kale, plus a starchy vegetable like carrots or potatoes; then add something filling like mushrooms, Brussels sprouts, or beans. This array, combined with a small salad, should do the trick. But if they don't have enough sides, or can't make them without pork, butter, or cheese, keep movin'.

STEP 4: Check out the sidekicks. This is another place that vegetables hang out. Most meat, fish, and poultry entrées come with a side dish. Whether the salmon is sautéed over Tuscan kale, or the chicken with roasted butternut squash, you can often take the latter part of these entrées and make a dish of them. Ask nicely, of course.

STEP 5: Eye the apps. Appetizers are typically written like food labels, from highest percent of ingredients to lowest. Meaning: The first thing listed makes up the bulk of the dish, and the last ingredient is usually a garnish. So if the first or second ingredient in the description is plant-based, you can usually remove the bacon or cheese and enjoy.

STEP 6: Peek at the pizzas and pastas. If all else fails, head to the pasta/pizza section. It's never your first stop since it generally means a big bowl of starches, but you can use the strategies above to build your own. All you need to do is order with any vegetables that caught your eye. This may mean taking pasta with tomato sauce and adding peas, mushrooms, spinach, and basil (ask the waiter what vegetables are available that night). Or ordering a pizza with peppers, onions, mushrooms, spinach, tomatoes, broccoli, basil, and tomato sauce. Don't be afraid to be creative by ordering whatever the restaurant clearly has in the back—but also remember to be overly kind, polite, and thankful for them accommodating.

How to Communicate with Your Server

Living with any dietary restriction, be it gluten-free, dairy-free, egg-free, nut-free, animal-free, nightshade-free, sugar-free, or [fill in the blank]-free, can make mealtime anything but stress-free. It's one thing to prepare your food at home, where you have the ability to plan, shop, cook, and control every bite. But going out is a whole other ball game. When you eat in a restaurant, the entire fate of your meal rests in the hands of your server. Think of them as the telephone line to the people preparing your food—that line can carry a static-y message ("Can you hear me now?"), drop the call entirely, or have a crystal-clear connection with the kitchen. The good news is communicating with a server is an art that can be mastered.

Here are some tips based on my years of experience as both a server and a cook:

1. Specify. Don't ever just expect your server knows what any of these phrases mean. He might think vegans can eat butter. He might think couscous is gluten-free. He might not know a nightshade from a lampshade.

Be specific. Tell him exactly what you are avoiding: butter, cheese, tomatoes, wheat, etc. Double-check that your specific ingredient is not in the dish you are ordering. If he seems doubtful, ask him politely to check with the kitchen. Just don't ever assume you're on the same page; put yourself on the same page.

2. Be creative, but not too creative. Often it proves more effective to modify an existing menu item than to create your own. (An exception is if you're in a high-end restaurant where there's a brilliant and passionate chef in the back eager to improvise.) For the most part, you'll be dealing with skilled cooks who are trained in the dishes on the menu. So order the item that requires the least changes—the pasta with olive oil to replace the cream sauce, the salad with chickpeas instead of the bacon, the burger without the bun. Think outside the box, but stay inside the menu.

3. Ask and then ask again. Never assume a dressing is made without eggs or a soup without cream or a veggie burger without corn. Ask about everything you're thinking of getting, because there's nothing worse than ordering a meal, getting it delivered chock-full of cheese, and sending it back because *you* forgot to ask to hold the Parmesan.

4. Study up. If you have dietary restrictions that go beyond "No butter, please," do a little pre-dining research. Before you journey over to a restaurant, check out the menu online to make sure you'll have something to eat. Try to find three options, just in case there's a hidden forbidden ingredient in one or two.

5. Get graphic. I used to feel that sometimes you need to say that you have an *allergy* to butter, peppers, or flour to make sure your needs are met. But then I got backlash from servers who said that when the word "allergy" is used, they have to have a rigmarole of special cutting boards and knives to make sure they don't get slapped with a lawsuit if you get a dab of butter. This made me feel bad about lying about my non-deadly allergies, so now I have a different tactic: I get graphic. I tell the server, point blank, "Please cook that spinach in oil, not butter. I can't have dairy. If they use butter by mistake instead, I will be so sick and I'd rather sleep in my bed than on my toilet tonight." That gets the point across.

6. Be oh-so kind. Some servers are wonderfully accommodating to restricted eaters. Perhaps they can relate because they themselves or their loved one has a unique dietary need, or they're an understanding person, or maybe they just want a big tip. Others are difficult to work and communicate with. Perhaps their ex had a dietary restriction that they're still bitter about, or they lack sensitivity and patience, or they're nervous because they've never gotten this request before, or they just want to leave work early. Whoever you get, always treat them with kindness. Being polite, appreciative, and grateful can truly make the difference between your server going above and beyond to help you eat a fantastic meal and your server telling you the house salad is your only option. "Please" and "thank you" go a long way.

WHAT TO MAKE WHEN YOU WANNA WIN THE BAKE SALE!

I don't know if bake sales are still a thing (can you use Venmo at a bake sale?), but my desire to win is forever. So whether you're trying to get top prize or just win someone's affection, you can count on these cookies to get the job done without getting your body mad.

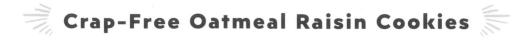

Crap-Free Oatmeal Raisin Cookies

Oatmeal raisin cookies made me realize I was marrying my father. Once, in a bakery with more treats than true crime docs on Netflix, I watched both men in my life beeline to the oatmeal raisins. I learned that a) therapy might be wise and b) I must create an outstanding oatmeal raisin cookie that I felt fab about my guys enjoying. This is that recipe, which is husband-approved, father-approved, and body-approved since it's oil-free, refined sugar–free, egg-free, dairy-free, and gluten-free.

MAKES 12 TO 14 COOKIES

DRY INGREDIENTS

½ cup almond flour (or meal)

1½ cups rolled oats (certified gluten-free if needed, not the quick-cooking ones)

½ teaspoon cinnamon

¼ teaspoon baking soda

⅛ teaspoon sea salt or pink salt

⅓ cup coconut sugar

½ cup raisins (or sub chocolate chips!)

WET INGREDIENTS

⅓ cup almond butter (or cashew, peanut, or sunflower butter)

2 tablespoons maple syrup or honey

¼ cup plain, unsweetened almond milk

½ teaspoon vanilla extract

1. Preheat the oven to 350°F.
2. In a large bowl, combine the almond flour, oats, cinnamon, baking soda, salt, coconut sugar, and raisins.
3. In a small bowl, combine the nut butter, maple syrup, almond milk, and vanilla. Whisk the wet stuff together.
4. Pour the wet ingredients into the dry ingredients and mix well.
5. Line a baking sheet with parchment paper.
6. Use your hands to form the batter into balls. Place them on the baking sheet and use the bottom of your measuring cup to flatten them onto discs.
7. Bake for 12 minutes, until very lightly brown.
8. Let them cool for a couple of minutes and then enjoy.
9. Store leftovers airtight on the counter.

HEALTHY EATING SUCKS:

"They were way better than I expected. My very picky brother loved them. And he hates 'healthy food.'" **—SB**

[Coconut] Sugar Cut-Out Cookies

Cut-out cookies are the original emojis, expressing everything from "Happy Hanukkah!" to "I love you!" to "Yay laundry day!" (That's what those sock cookie cutter shapes are for, right?) Crunchy on the outside but so chewy and soft on the inside, these are my faves.

MAKES 10 TO 20ISH COOKIES, DEPENDING ON WHAT SHAPE AND SIZE YOU CUT THEM INTO

2 cups almond flour (a.k.a. almond meal)

½ teaspoon baking powder

¼ teaspoon salt

⅓ cup coconut sugar

1 teaspoon vanilla extract

½ teaspoon lemon extract

2 tablespoon refined coconut oil, melted, plus a smidge more for painting on

¼ cup maple syrup

Festive sprinkles of your choosing

1. Mix the almond flour, baking powder, salt, and coconut sugar together and remove any almond flour lumps, then mix the vanilla, lemon extract, coconut oil, and maple syrup right into the bowl.

2. Mix together really well, using your hands if necessary, then roll into a ball and cover with plastic wrap. Plop that into your fridge for about 40 minutes (watch a third of your favorite movie!?).

3. Preheat the oven to 350°F. Line a baking sheet with parchment paper.

4. Remove the dough from the fridge and roll out. The thinner you roll, the crispier the cookies will be.

5. Cut the rolled dough with your favorite cookie cutters and place on the prepared baking sheet.

6. "Paint" on some melted coconut oil—if you don't have a brush just use your fingers or a spoon—and then decorate with sprinkles.

7. Bake for 12 to 17 minutes (the thinner the cookies, the less time), until lightly golden.

8. Let sit to harden for a bit and enjoy.

CBD! EASY AS ABC!

Baking with CBD is an easy-as-ABC way to get more of the lovely hemp plant–derived supplement without holding the herbal tasting oil straight under your tongue for 30 seconds. Famous for its anti-inflammatory and anti-anxiety properties without the "Wait, why is my dog reciting Shakespeare?" properties CBD can be a cool way to calm down and is best used frequently so its effects compound. That means that adding it to your cookies makes your cookies something best eaten frequently, so you are welcome. I sometimes like to add 1 to 2 teaspoons of CBD oil to my cookies, brownies, or snack balls to make them extra fun for my insides.

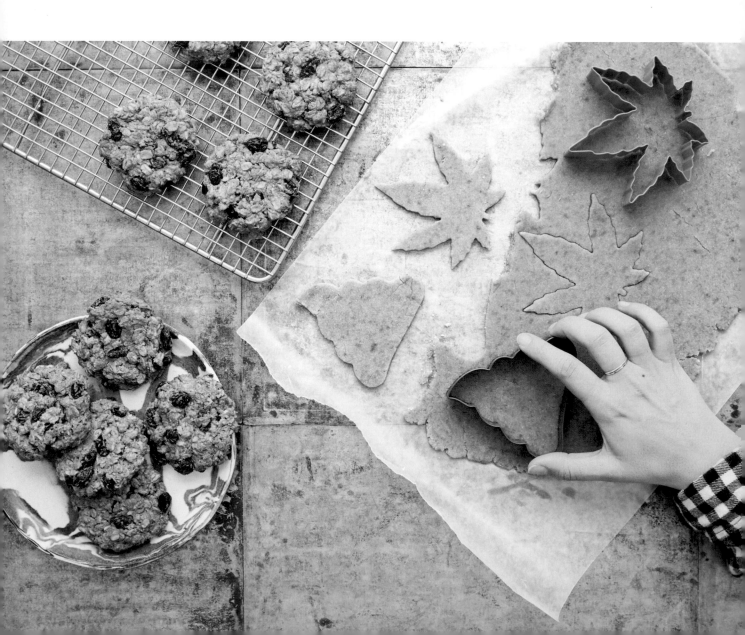

WHEN YOU WANNA SNEAK A SNACK INTO THE MOVIES (OR ONTO YOUR COUCH)

I can't remember the last time I bought butter-drenched movie theater popcorn. Maybe around the time I printed out directions on MapQuest to get to the theater? Since I started making this easy homemade version, which you can eat by the bucket with no guilt and no bellyache, I've never gone back. Salt and nutritional yeast are my go-to toppings, but the sweet and spicy combination of mango plus sriracha and the cinnamon kettle corn with chocolate make even the worst movies enjoyable.

Super-Fun Mango Sriracha Popcorn Mix

SERVES 2 GOOD SHARERS

4 teaspoons coconut oil, butter-flavored if desired

½ teaspoon sea salt

1 tablespoon sriracha

½ cup organic popcorn kernels

¼ to ½ cup dried mango, coarsely chopped

1. Melt 1 teaspoon of the coconut oil in a small saucepan over medium-low heat. Remove from the heat and add the salt and sriracha. Set aside.

2. In a large pot over medium-low to medium heat, melt the remaining 3 teaspoons coconut oil.

3. When the oil's melted and the pot seems hot, toss 1 popcorn kernel in; if the oil sizzles, you're good to go.

4. Dump in all of the kernels, put on the lid, and begin shaking the pot over the burner. Soon, you'll hear popping! Once the sound of pops are slow and far apart, turn off the heat and dump your popped popcorn into a large bowl.

5. Add the sriracha mixture and use your hands to toss it all around so it spreads evenly.

6. Add the dried mango and use your hands to mix it around.

7. Can be stored in a resealable plastic baggie or glass jar to be eaten later.

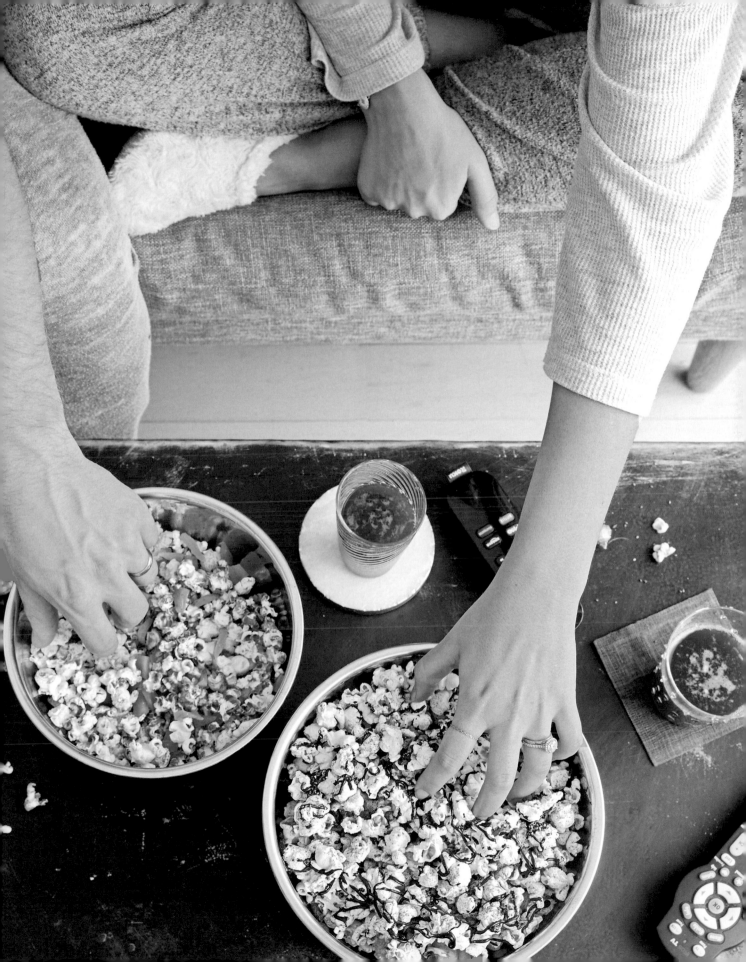

Decked-Out Cinnamon Kettle Corn

1 teaspoon sea salt

Cinnamon to taste

3 tablespoons coconut sugar

4 teaspoons coconut oil

½ cup organic popcorn kernels

Coconut oil spray (optional)

TO DECK IT OUT

¼ cup "Sexy Can I Drizzle This Magic Chocolate Sauce" (page 79) and/or:

¼ cup drizzly peanut butter or almond butter (If your nut butter is on the firmer side, mix it in a small dish with 1 tablespoon melted coconut oil and 1 tablespoon maple syrup, then use a fork to drizzle on your popcorn.)

Chia seeds, more cinnamon, salt, cacao nibs, chocolate chips, or sprinkles

1. In a small bowl, mix the salt, cinnamon, and coconut sugar together and set aside.

2. In a large pot over medium-low to medium heat, melt 3 teaspoons of the coconut oil.

3. When the oil's melted and the pot seems hot, toss 1 popcorn kernel in the pot; if the oil fizzles, you're good to go.

4. Dump in all the kernels, put on the lid, and begin shaking the pot over the burner. Soon, you'll hear popping! Once the sound of pops are slow and far apart, turn off the heat and dump your popped popcorn into a large bowl.

5. If you have coconut oil spray, spray it all over your popcorn to give it a sticky coat to help the salt/cinnamon/sugar mixture stick. If you don't, melt the remaining 1 teaspoon coconut oil and use your hands to mix it in.

6. Add the salt/cinnamon/sugar mixture to the popcorn and use your hands to toss it all around so it spreads evenly. Add your optional toppings.

7. Can be stored in a resealable baggie or glass jar to be eaten later.

WHEN YOU'RE SIPPING FROM YOUR THERMOS

Before almond milk hit every coffee shop on the planet, I used to feel like such a sad sack every time latte season struck. By the time the nondairy trend came around and I could order from a barista without a bellyache, I'd already perfected the art of making my own lattes. Sorrynotsorry, Starbucks!

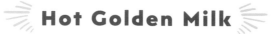

Hot Golden Milk

Originally a holistic Indian Ayurvedic bevvie, my riff on this golden beauty will rock your modern world. It isn't just eye-catching or shirt-staining (you've been warned!) but it's rich in antioxidants and anti-inflammatory compounds thanks to the ingredients behind that healthy hue: turmeric and ginger. Add to them the brown trio of nutmeg, cinnamon, and cardamom and it makes sense where those claims of being gut-soothing, relaxation-inducing, and inflammation-healing fame come from.

MAKES 1 MUG

1 cup plain, unsweetened almond milk or other nondairy milk

¼ teaspoon vanilla extract

½ teaspoon ground turmeric

¼ teaspoon cardamom

¼ teaspoon ground ginger

¼ teaspoon cinnamon

Pinch of nutmeg

Pinch of freshly ground black pepper

1½ teaspoons coconut sugar or another sweetener, such as a Medjool date, 1 teaspoon organic cane or palm sugar, honey, maple syrup, or stevia to taste

1. Place the almond milk, vanilla, turmeric, cardamom, ginger, cinnamon, nutmeg, pepper, and coconut sugar into a blender and blend until frothy.

2. Pour into a small pot on the stove over medium to medium-high heat. Heat to a light boil, then reduce the heat and simmer for about 1 minute.

3. Pour into a mug and sip or slurp.

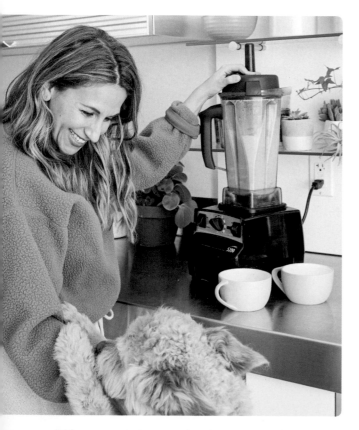

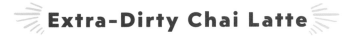

Extra-Dirty Chai Latte

When *The Dr. Oz Show* asked me to create a recipe that could take coffee to new, healthier heights, I conceived of this Extra-Dirty Chai Latte (pictured on page 126). This latte has almost too many health benefits for just one drink. First, the espresso provides clean energy and antioxidants. Then, the warming spices like cardamom, ginger, and cinnamon work in tandem to nourish your body. (These particular spices have been used medicinally for centuries for their cleansing and digestion-boosting properties.) Mushroom powder is one of the most potent and powerful superfoods on the planet. And without dairy or processed sugar, you can rest easy knowing every ingredient is health supportive rather than destructive.

MAKES 1 MUG

1½ cups plain, unsweetened almond, oat, or other plant milk

1 organic chai tea bag

1 shot of espresso

1½ teaspoons maple syrup

1½ teaspoons mushroom powder (I recommend Cordyceps for energy, Lions Mane for mental clarity, and Chaga for extra antioxidants)

⅛ teaspoon vanilla extract

⅛ teaspoon cinnamon

Pinch of cardamom (optional)

Pinch of ginger (optional)

1. In a small saucepan, simmer the almond milk with the chai tea bag. Whisk the bag around a little so you start to see the almond milk darken, then remove it from the heat. Discard the tea bag.

2. Place the almond milk in a blender and add the espresso, maple syrup, mushroom powder, vanilla, cinnamon, and cardamom and ginger, if using. Blend until everything is combined. This will help your latte froth up, coffee shop style.

3. Pour into a mug and enjoy.

AFTER [PARTY] THOUGHT:

Want it less dirty? Nix the espresso and enjoy
a warming mushroom chai latte.

Anything but Basic PSL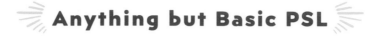

I'm not always up with the lingo so when my friend said the pumpkin spice latte I had whipped up was "basic," I responded with an earnest, "Not really, I mean, this one uses real pumpkin, which I don't think the coffee shops do." I then learned there was an alternative meaning of "basic," which has been weaponized against PSLs, which is stupid because PSLs are basically amazing and no one should be shamed for enjoying them.

MAKES 1 MUG

1 cup plain, unsweetened almond milk

3 tablespoons pumpkin puree

¼ teaspoon pumpkin pie spice, plus more as a garnish

¼ teaspoon cinnamon

¼ teaspoon vanilla extract

Pinch of sea salt or pink salt

Stevia or maple syrup to taste

1. Pulse the almond milk, pumpkin puree, pumpkin pie spice, cinnamon, vanilla, and salt six times in a blender.
2. Transfer the mixture to a small pot on the stove and heat up to your desired temperature.
3. Once warm enough for you, pour into a mug and sweeten to your liking.
4. Garnish with a sprinkle of pumpkin pie spice if you're fancy.

AFTER [PARTY] THOUGHT:

CRAZY ABOUT COFFEE? Add a shot of espresso to this latte and you'll love it even more.

WHEN IT'S BEACH DAY, OR YOU'RE PICNICKING IN THE PARK 'CUZ YOU'RE CUTE LIKE THAT

Filling your cooler with not-good beach food is not cool. When it comes to packing for the beach, nutritious food that packs well and tastes good is way more important than a sun umbrella that runs a 79 percent risk of getting swept up by the wind and impaling your neighbor. This is why I took the curation of these recipes extra seriously, and why these three recipes are extra spectacular.

Muhammara May I

Is it a dip? A spread? A sunscreen? Muhammara is a zesty, peppery Middle Eastern dish that makes hummus feel the way I feel when I go down the rabbit hole of Instagram influencers—less good about myself in comparison. Traditionally a combination of roasted red peppers and walnuts, my version adds white beans so that eating it really satisfies.

MAKES A LOT!

1 heaping cup roasted red bell peppers (you can find them in jars packed in water)

2 tablespoons olive oil

2 garlic cloves, chopped

1 tablespoon honey or maple syrup

1 tablespoon freshly squeezed lemon juice

1 teaspoon cumin

½ teaspoon chili powder

¼ to ½ teaspoon sea salt or pink salt

Pinch of cayenne if you like things spicy

1 15-ounce can great northern beans or cannellini beans (a.k.a. white beans)

⅓ cup raw walnuts, raw pumpkin seeds, or raw sunflower seeds

1. Combine the peppers, olive oil, garlic, honey, lemon juice, cumin, chili powder, salt, cayenne, beans, and walnuts in a blender or food processor and process until smooth. You might need to pause, scrape down the sides, and then process some more.

2. This is a super spread for veggie-loaded sandwiches as well as a bomb-diggity dip for crackers and crunchy veggies.

3. Store leftovers in a sealed container in the fridge.

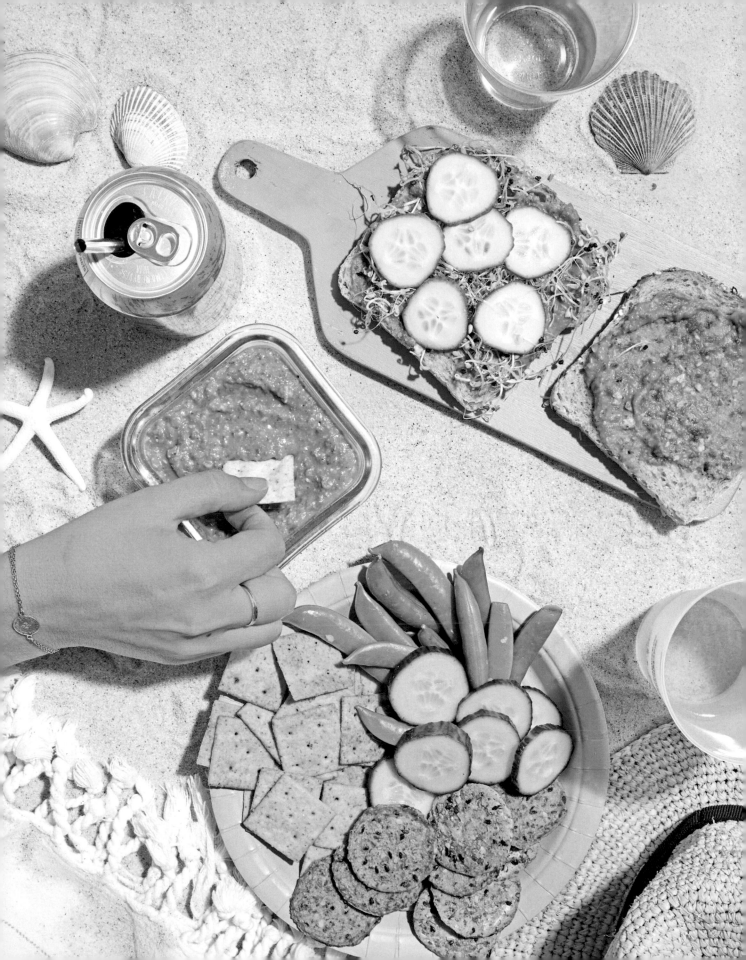

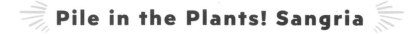

Pile in the Plants! Sangria

If *Party in My Plants* had a theme song, it would be this sangria. It embodies the entirety of my eating ethos: It's fun, simple, energizing, portable, refreshing, vibrant, party-pleasing, cute, sweet, spunky, approachable, luscious, and giggle-inducing. It's also slightly dangerous. For example, during the photo shoot for this recipe, what you don't see is how much sangria is in my belly. Because I couldn't stop drinking it in between takes. This is also how I learned that consuming this sangria like a soup is swell.

MAKES A PITCHER OF 4 TO 6 DRINKS

1 cup watermelon or pineapple, chopped

1 green apple, cored and chopped

1 pear or peach, cored or pitted and chopped

1 orange, peeled and chopped

1 lime, peeled and chopped

1 bottle of white wine or rosé

2 to 3 tablespoons maple syrup or agave to taste (optional)

2 to 3 tablespoons fresh mint, plus more for garnish

3 to 4 cups ice

1. In a large pitcher (a portable one if you're taking it to go), combine the watermelon, apple, pear, orange, lime, wine, maple syrup, if using, mint, and ice. Use a long spoon to mix it all together.

2. Chill in your fridge for 30 minutes and garnish with a sprig of mint.

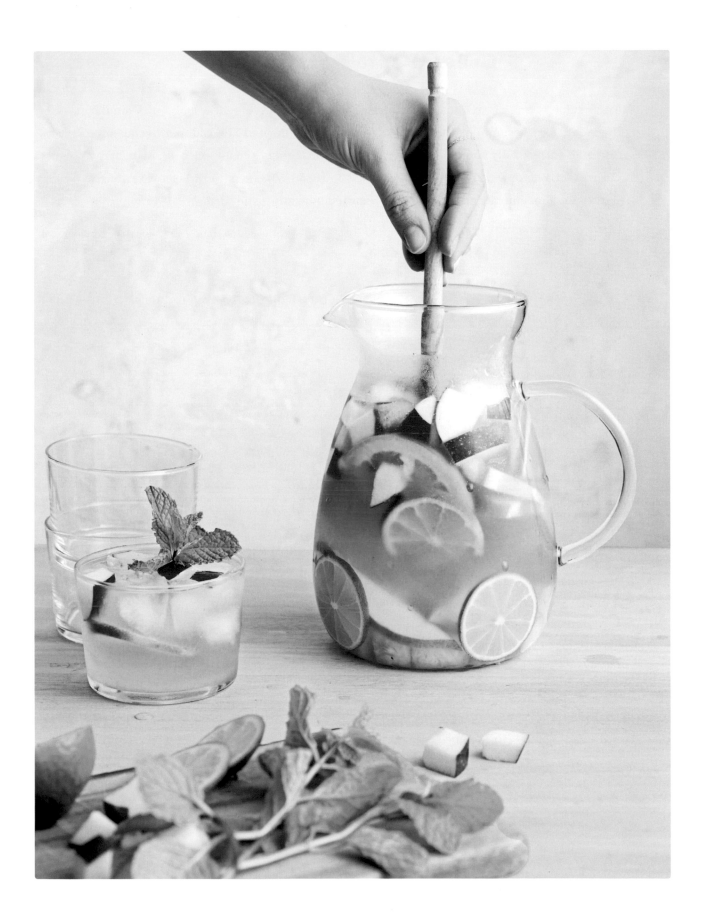

Greek Pasta Party Salad

This recipe is one of my most prized possessions. After I created it, I was in a similar mental state (I assume) as the person was when they created The Clapper because we had both successfully combined two f*%ing fabulous things. (Pasta + Greek Salad, in my case. Light + clapping in Joseph Pedott's case in 1985.) What's extra rad is it is seriously party-sized, meaning it makes like nine hundred portions.

SERVES 8 TO 10 (HALVING WORKS—AS DO LEFTOVERS)

SALAD

12 to 16 ounces your favorite dry pasta in your favorite shape (I love a lentil or chickpea or brown rice pasta in macaroni or fusilli shape)

1 large cucumber, peeled and chopped small

1 pint cherry tomatoes, cut into quarters

1 cup kalamata olives, pitted and cut in half

1 small or ½ large red onion, diced small

1 bell pepper of your choosing, diced small

1 15-ounce can of chickpeas, drain and rinsed (optional)

Your favorite dairy-free cheese or feta cheese (1 to 2 cups small chunks or about 7 to 14 ounces)

Fresh parsley, to taste (optional)

DRESSING

3 or 4 garlic cloves, chopped

¼ cup freshly squeezed lemon juice (about 1 large lemon)

5 tablespoons apple cider vinegar (if you're not into vinegar, use 3 tablespoons)

½ to 2 teaspoons sea salt (This will vary depending on how much/what kind of cheese you're adding. Start with ½ teaspoon, dress the salad, taste, and add more salt as needed.)

¼ to ½ teaspoon freshly ground black pepper, plus more to taste

2 teaspoons dried oregano, plus more to taste

½ cup extra-virgin olive oil

PRO TIP:

Make this the night before a party so the flavors marinate and taste even better.

1. Cook the pasta al dente, according to the package instructions.

2. Once your pasta is cooked, drain and let it sit in the colander to dry. Transfer to a big salad bowl.

3. Add the cucumber, tomatoes, olives, onion, bell pepper, chickpeas, cheese, and parsley, if using, and mix well to make sure they're dispersed throughout.

4. To make the dressing, in a blender add the garlic, lemon juice, vinegar, salt, pepper, and oregano. Then slowly add the olive oil.

5. Dress your salad, mix it really well, and add additional seasoning (oregano, black pepper, salt) to taste.

6. Keep in the fridge until it's ready to serve.

7. Store leftovers in the fridge.

LEFTOVERS ARE THE BESTOVERS:

Eat over fresh greens or put some into a wrap as a meal.

HEALTHY EATING SUCKS:

"My fiancé, who usually bitches about meatless meals, loved it and was complaining about how full he was after. WIN!" —MH

AFTER [PARTY] THOUGHT:

Take your picnic on a hike! One recipe tester said: "I ate that shiz cold out of a Tupperware *and* took it on a climbing/camping trip to share with friends. It kept in a cooler super well and tasted great. People were pumped to have real food on a climbing trip for once." —DC

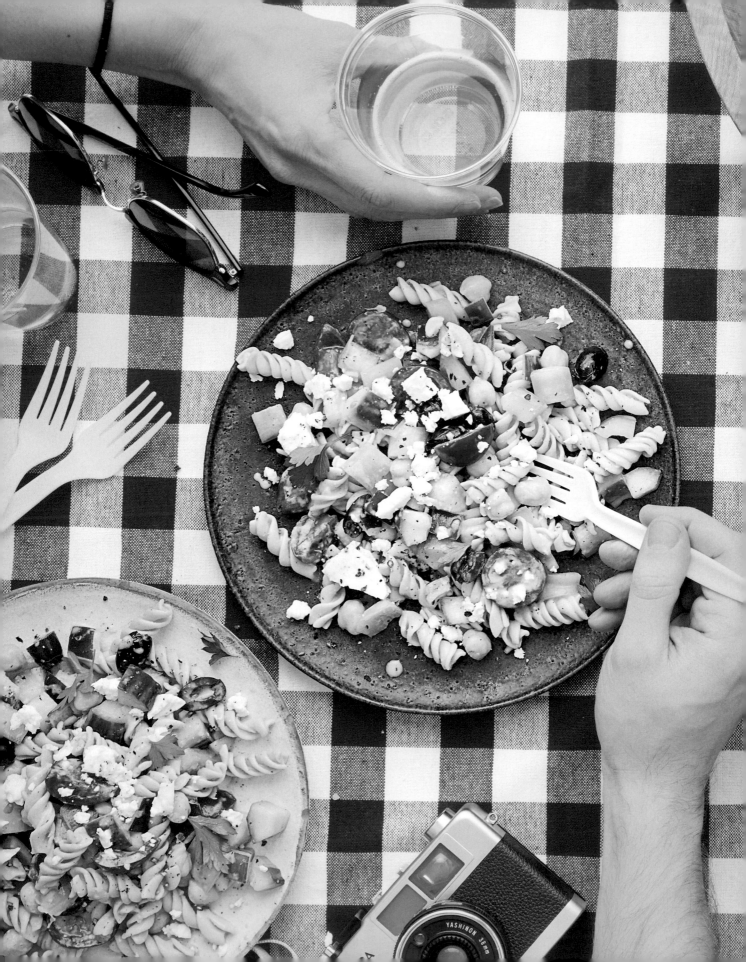

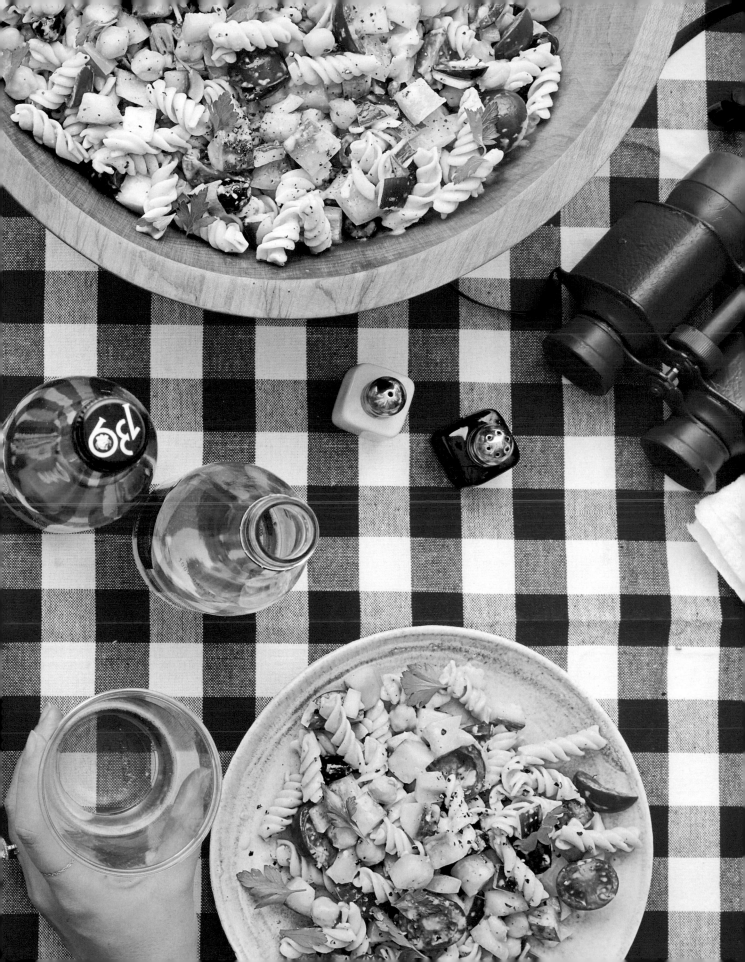

WHAT TO MAKE WHEN YOU'RE TAILGATING, OTHERWISE KNOWN AS EATING IN A PARKING LOT

Having been raised by a father from Pittsburgh, following football is in my blood—and pregaming in parking lots was in my OkCupid profile list of hobbies. My uncle even has Steelers season tickets, which we lovingly mooch as much as we can. Tailgates were always peak "high-maintenance-healthy loser," as I had to awkwardly ask Uncle Herky if we could stop at Whole Foods en route to the game so I could get "Talia food." It took me years of "there's gotta be a better way than eating my own cubed pineapple in 30-degree weather that I grabbed because it was sitting by the register and I felt guilty holding everyone up" to realize that what I needed to do was bring these recipes instead. Eventually, everyone started asking when I'd be bringing out the kombucha cocktails, buffalo dip, and blondies.

There's an "I" in Buffalo Cauliflower Dip

We can thank both FOMO and my personal dislike of artichokes for this recipe. Whether it was a tailgate, Super Bowl party, or non-sport-focused gathering, I'd gotten sick of standing to the side when my hostess brought a bubbling, creamy buffalo dip hot outta the oven. Then, one year when Jesse and I were hosting Friendsgiving, my friend Ilene debuted a kale artichoke dip[9] that was dairy-free-for-me—and I realized that not even that could make me love artichokes. So I got to work creating a hybrid that hits the spot.

SERVES 8 TO 10 AT A PARTY (HALVE THE RECIPE IF YOU WANT TO SERVE LESS)

½ cup raw cashews, soaked for at least 30 minutes in warm water

1 large head of cauliflower

3 tablespoons olive oil

Sea salt and freshly ground black pepper to taste

2 to 3 large garlic cloves

½ yellow onion

6 cups kale

1 15-ounce can white or cannellini beans, drained and rinsed

1 15-ounce can full-fat coconut milk

Juice of ½ a lemon (about 1 tablespoon lemon juice)

2 tablespoons nutritional yeast

5 ounces (⅔ cup) Frank's RedHot sauce

Crackers, chips, or celery sticks for serving and scooping

1. Soak the cashews in a bowl with enough warm or hot water to cover them fully for at least 30 minutes.
2. Preheat the oven to 425°F.
3. Chop, wash, and dry the cauliflower. You want to chop it into small florets or chunks. Think bite-size or scoopable-size.
4. Add the cauliflower to a large bowl and toss with 2 tablespoons of the olive oil plus a generous sprinkle of sea salt and pepper. Mix it so the cauliflower gets coated evenly, then transfer it to a rimmed baking sheet lined with aluminum foil.
5. Roast for 20 minutes or until lightly golden brown. Flip the cauliflower after 10 minutes for even roasting.

continued

9. Which is in her cookbook called *The Colorful Kitchen!* Plant party approved.

6. While the cauliflower is roasting, chop the garlic, onion, and kale and set aside.

7. When the cauliflower is done, remove it from the oven and set aside. Reduce the oven temperature to 400°F.

8. In a high-speed blender, add the beans, coconut milk, lemon juice, nutritional yeast, drained and rinsed cashews, and hot sauce. Blend until creamy. Set aside.

9. Heat the remaining 1 tablespoon olive oil in a large cast-iron skillet over medium-high heat. Add the onion and garlic and sauté for about 5 minutes, until the onion is translucent. Reduce the heat, add the kale, and sauté for 2 to 3 minutes, until the kale wilts and cooks down. Remove from the heat.

10. Add the cauliflower and spread it out in the skillet. Pour the blended mixture on top, using a spoon or spatula so everything's thoroughly combined and spread evenly.

11. Bake the whole shebang in the oven until the top is lightly brown, about 20 minutes.

12. Remove from the oven and let sit for about 10 minutes before serving with crackers, chips, or celery sticks.

13. Store any leftovers covered in the fridge and reheat in the oven.

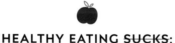

HEALTHY EATING SUCKS:

"This is a 10 out of 10 and I'm bringing it to every party for the rest of my life. My co-workers loved this and I'm pretty sure I convinced them all to buy your cookbook just so they have this recipe." **—AS**

 NOTE: Don't sweat it if you don't have a cast-iron skillet; sauté in a regular skillet and then transfer your mixture to an oven-safe baking dish for baking and serving.

Go Blondies

These superstar treats are a less tan version of my Fooled Ya Black Bean Brownies (page 279). Like how those stealthily sub black beans for flour, eggs, and oil for that ooey-gooey-ness we all love, their golden cousins utilize high-protein chickpeas. They're fun to deck out in vanilla frosting and festive sprinkles to match your team colors (or scream Happy Birthday! Happy Valentine's Day! Merry Secretary Day!) but they're obsession-inducing even naked.

SERVING SIZE DEPENDS ON HOW LARGE OR SMALL YOU CUT THEM

1 15-ounce can chickpeas, drained and rinsed

⅔ cup unsalted nut butter of choice (I recommend almond butter)

⅔ cup coconut sugar or organic cane sugar

1 teaspoon baking powder

2 teaspoon vanilla extract

¼ teaspoon sea salt

Sprinkles (optional)

½ to 1 cup chocolate chips

Coconut oil spray, for greasing the pan

Crap-Free Vanilla Frosting (page 146) (optional)

1. Preheat the oven to 350°F. Spray an 8 x 8-inch or 9 x 9-inch baking pan with coconut oil spray (or line it with parchment paper).
2. Place the chickpeas, nut butter, coconut sugar, baking powder, vanilla, and salt in a food processor and process away. You might need to pause and scrape down the sides and process again.
3. Once well combined, transfer the batter to a large bowl and mix in the sprinkles, if using, and chocolate chips.
4. Place the batter in the prepared pan, spreading it out evenly.
5. Bake for 27 to 30 minutes. Test to see if it's done by sticking a fork or knife in it (while it's in the oven). If it comes out clean, they're ready.
6. Remove from the oven and let it sit for about 15 minutes.
7. OPTIONAL = Frost with vanilla frosting and then add sprinkles on top.
8. Cut into whatever size blondies you want. Store leftovers sealed in a container in the fridge.

NOTE: You can freeze these blonde friends, too, for future NEED A BLONDIEMERGENCIES!

HEALTHY EATING SUCKS:

"My husband loved them and was mad that I put some aside in the freezer so he couldn't eat them." —AB

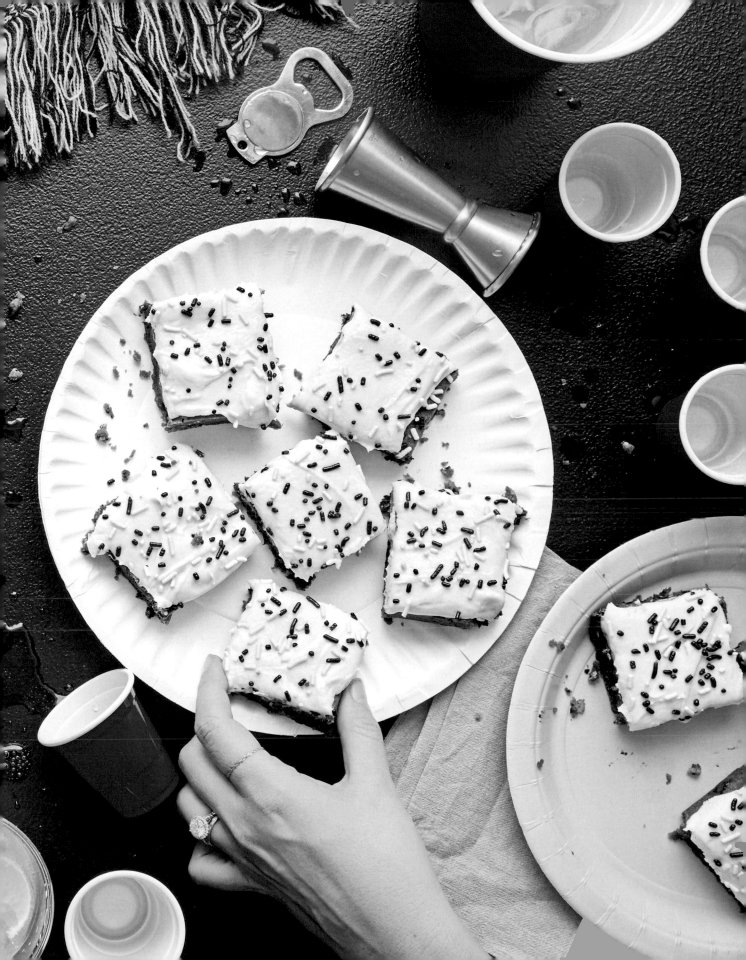

TOX WHILE YOU DETOX WITH KOMBUCHA COCKTAILS

Just because I like to party with plants doesn't mean I don't like to party . . . with other things. Like alcohol. (Which is really just fermented plants.)

Health and happiness go together. They *need* each other to maximize their individual potential. And what's something that enhances happiness for many of us? Alcohol. (In moderation.) I'm not suggesting spiking all of your cold-pressed juices. I just want you to know that, if you have an occasional drink to kick back, celebrate life, and giggle a little bit extra, you can do that without compromising your health.

I do this by making "Tox While I Detox" cocktails—which is a cute way of saying that I mix vodka or tequila with kombucha instead of soda or juice.

Why vodka or tequila?

The lighter the spirit, the lighter impact on your blood sugar and waistline. My go-to vodkas, which are both gluten-free, are Ciroc, which is distilled from grapes (like wine), and Tito's, which is distilled from corn (like tacos).

Why Kombucha?

If you don't know kombucha (apart from "that weird drink that once exploded all over my friend's car"), it's a beverage fermented from black tea and a little bit of sugar. It contains a SCOBY, which is made of bacteria and yeast, and which reacts with the sugar to birth an abundance of great-for-you microbes, alive and packed with enzymes, which means that kombucha has tremendous nutritional value.

THOSE SUPER-FLY LIVE ENZYMES:

DETOXIFY US.

The enzymes and probiotics (yes, like the supplements your doctor recommends) in kombucha kick ass at detoxifying our guts. The more good bacteria, the better and quicker we get rid of the bad stuff, so drinking kombucha can speed up that whole process. This also helps with liver function.

BOOST OUR IMMUNE SYSTEM.

Strengthening our gut also works wonders for our immunity. Unfortunately, all those antibiotics or medications we take when we get sick wipe out the good bacteria in our bellies. Without good bacteria in our bellies, our immune system, which largely resides in our gut, is compromised. Fermented drinks help rebuild our microscopic buddies, and thus strengthen our immunity.

GIVE US B-VITS.

Kombucha contains B vitamins, which are mostly found in animals and thus can be a source of concern for plant-partiers. B vitamins help reduce stress, anxiety, depression, and PMS. They boost energy, heart, hair, skin, nails, and memory health. Kombucha isn't a replacement for a B-vitamin supplement (or eating a little fish or eggs every now and again), but it can give you a nice bonus.

GIVE US A LITTLE BUZZ.

A few years back, kombucha brewers were forced to put a 21+ label on their bottles, as some were found to contain at least .5% alcohol per bottle. Yes, just like how grapes are fermented into wine with big-time booze, kombucha has a minuscule amount of alcohol as well. (Not enough to get you a DUI if you drink it post-yoga but enough to give you a jolt of energy without the chemicals in most energy drinks.)

HAS A DELIGHTFUL FIZZ.

Kombucha builds up carbonation when it sits in an airtight bottle for long enough. Just a little—making it the perfect substitute for alcohol or the soda or juice that you'd normally mix in.

IS A PERFECT ALCOHOL SUBSTITUTE THAT LOOKS PRETTY IN A WINEGLASS, BEER MUG, OR SOLO UP AND/OR THE PERFECT SODA OR JUICE SUBSTITUTE TO MIX WITH THAT ALCOHOL.

I am telling you, I've had to start bringing like a case of kombucha bottles to New Year's Eve parties and tailgates to accommodate all the skeptical patrons who fall in love with this combination and then want to steal my stuff.

1 shot of VODKA + 4 to 6 ounces of KOMBUCHA + a pinch or drop of STEVIA or agave (if desired for sweetness)— over ice

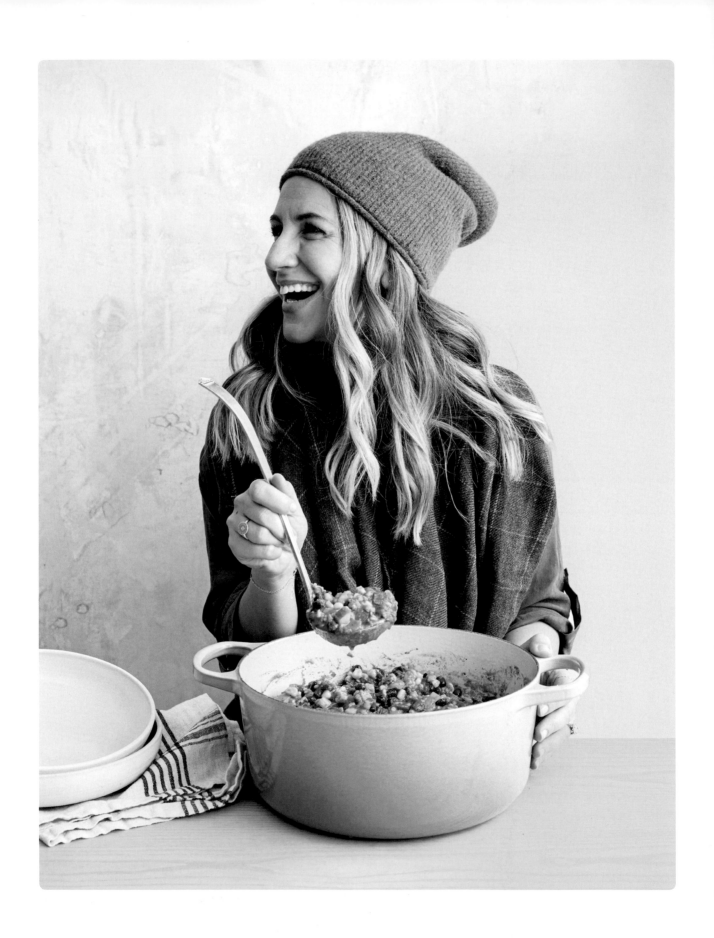

You'll TouchDOWN This Pumpkin Black Bean Chili

Everyone needs a go-to chili and this one is mine. It combines the coziest two things in the world (pumpkin and chili) in a one-pot meal that'll leave you satisfied for hours. With the black beans and tempeh, it packs a ton of fill-you-up protein, and the pumpkin pie spice, chili powder, and sage means it's a flavor explosion.

MAKES ABOUT 7 SMALL SERVINGS OR 4 HUGE ONES

2 tablespoons coconut oil or olive oil

1 sweet white onion, chopped

4 garlic cloves, minced

1 teaspoon salt, plus a few additional pinches

1 X-ounce package tempeh

1½ teaspoons chili powder

1 bell pepper (any color), diced

1 zucchini, chopped

1 15-ounce can pumpkin puree

1 28-ounce can diced tomatoes, with juice

½ teaspoon pumpkin pie spice

½ teaspoon dried sage

2 15-ounce cans black beans, drained and rinsed

1 cup frozen corn

Quinoa, brown rice, spread-eagle sweet potatoes, avocado chunks, tortilla chips, or hot sauce, for serving

1. In a large stockpot, add 1 tablespoon of the coconut oil and melt it over medium heat.

2. Once the oil is hot, add the onion and garlic and a pinch of salt.

3. Sauté for 3 to 5 minutes, until the onion becomes translucent and soft.

4. While the onion mixture is cooking, melt the remaining 1 tablespoon coconut oil in a sauté pan over medium heat.

5. Break up the package of tempeh with your fingers and add it to the pan. Mix in ½ teaspoon of the chili powder and a pinch of salt and sauté for 5 minutes, until a little browned.

6. While the tempeh cooks, go back to your stockpot and add the bell pepper. Sauté for a minute or two. Then add the zucchini and sauté for another minute.

7. Add the pumpkin puree, diced tomatoes with their juice, the remaining 1 teaspoon chili powder, the sage, the pumpkin pie spice, and the salt. Stir.

8. The tempeh should be perfectly cooked. Add it to the large pot and mix.

9. Add the black beans and the frozen corn and mix well.

10. Cover the pot and raise the heat to high and cook until the chili starts to boil.

11. Reduce the heat to a simmer and cook for 30 more minutes.

12. Serve over cooked quinoa, brown rice, or a spread-eagle sweet potato. Dress it up with chunks of avocado and a handful of crushed baked tortilla chips. If you like things extra hot, add some hot sauce.

AFTER [PARTY] THOUGHT:

If you're making this for someone who *must have meat*, consider splitting the finished product in two and adding cooked ground turkey to their portion. It's okay, they're still packing tons of plants into their bods.

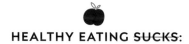

HEALTHY EATING ~~SUCKS~~:

"My friend, a carnivorous Midwestern boy who always makes fun of my 'weird vegan food,' ate two bowls and kept saying it tasted like fall in a bowl." —NRS

WHEN YOU'RE TRAVELING

Airplane travel often prompts some "Screw it, I'm gonna get dehydrated, hungry, gassy, and gross" behavior.

But to that I say, "WRONG 'TUDE, DUDE!"

When done right, airplane travel can be smooth sailing—I mean, smooth flying. The key is to focus on *protein*. Why? Because it'll fill you up, and keep you full, so you're not tempted to go for the $17 cheese plate the flight attendants are hawking.

TIP #1: Maybe even more annoying than a crying baby on a plane is the dehydration that sets in. To avoid landing as an exhausted, weak, cranky version of yourself, you gotta drink water. Because those wimpy cups they pass out ain't gonna cut it, BYO bottle and refill it every chance you get. Minimally, you want to guzzle 1 cup of water per hour. Peeing frequently means it's working, so do yourself a favor and get an aisle seat so you don't disturb your neighbors (or regret not wearing a diaper).

TIP #2: If an apple a day keeps the doctor away, an apple a flight keeps you feeling aiight. Apples are no-nonsense travel buddies; a fly-friendly fruit that doesn't spoil, bruise, leak, and ruin your iPad like *cough* bananas. My rule? Never pack a carry-on without one.

TIP #3: If you tend to be tempted by free snacks (no judgment—the snack cart's the most exciting thing going on up there), bring your own. Ziplocks of homemade popcorn, Curry Car Cashews (page 257), Cheeseisn'ts (page 88), snap peas or carrot and bell pepper sticks all make for better choices than the crap-in-a-bag you're likely to get.

TIP #4: When you're 30,000 feet up in the air and you get a craving for something sweet, there aren't many options. (*Unless you have a healthy lip gloss?*) I tote small bags of dried mangos, Bananagrams (page 258), Very Present-able Pecans (page 260), or Snickerdoodlerolls (page 255) to satisfy my in-flight craving.

TIP #5: Carry on a meal. Prepare it at home and pop it in your bag or get takeout from your fave spot on the way to the airport. For a very long flight, bring an insulated lunch box with an icepack or two.

The "Too Good to Have a Fear of Heights" Green Sandie

It was once shocking to type a credit card number into a computer and now it's arguably way too normal. Likewise, it was once shocking for me to see this sandwich on a breakfast menu and now I eat it all the time when I'm at that specific breakfast place.[10] Granted, it was the only planty, non-eggy thing I could eat on said breakfast menu, but thank all the sprouts and fairies for that because now this sandwich can make its way into your life. It's perfect for travel because it's nonperishable (within reason); easily transportable; and TSA-friendly; it's filling from the avocado, nut butter, and fiber-rich sprouted bun; and it's nutritious from the kale.

MAKES 1 SANDWICH

1 teaspoon olive oil

1 garlic clove, minced

2 cups kale, chopped, rinsed, and ribs removed

Pinch of sea salt or pink salt

1 sprouted-grain, whole-wheat, or gluten-free English muffin

¼ medium avocado

1 tablespoon almond butter

1. Heat the olive oil in a sauté pan over medium heat. Add the garlic and sauté for about 2 minutes.
2. Add the kale and a pinch of salt and sauté for about 5 minutes, until slightly crispy.
3. While the kale is sautéing, toast the English muffin.
4. Mash the avocado onto one side of the English muffin and spread almond butter on the other side.
5. Layer the cooked kale and, well, make a sandwich.
6. Enjoy now or wrap up in aluminum foil for in-flight entertainment.

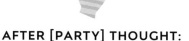

AFTER [PARTY] THOUGHT:

If you or your other half eats fried eggs,
I hear it's delightful to add one.

10. Shout out to the Green on Nantucket!

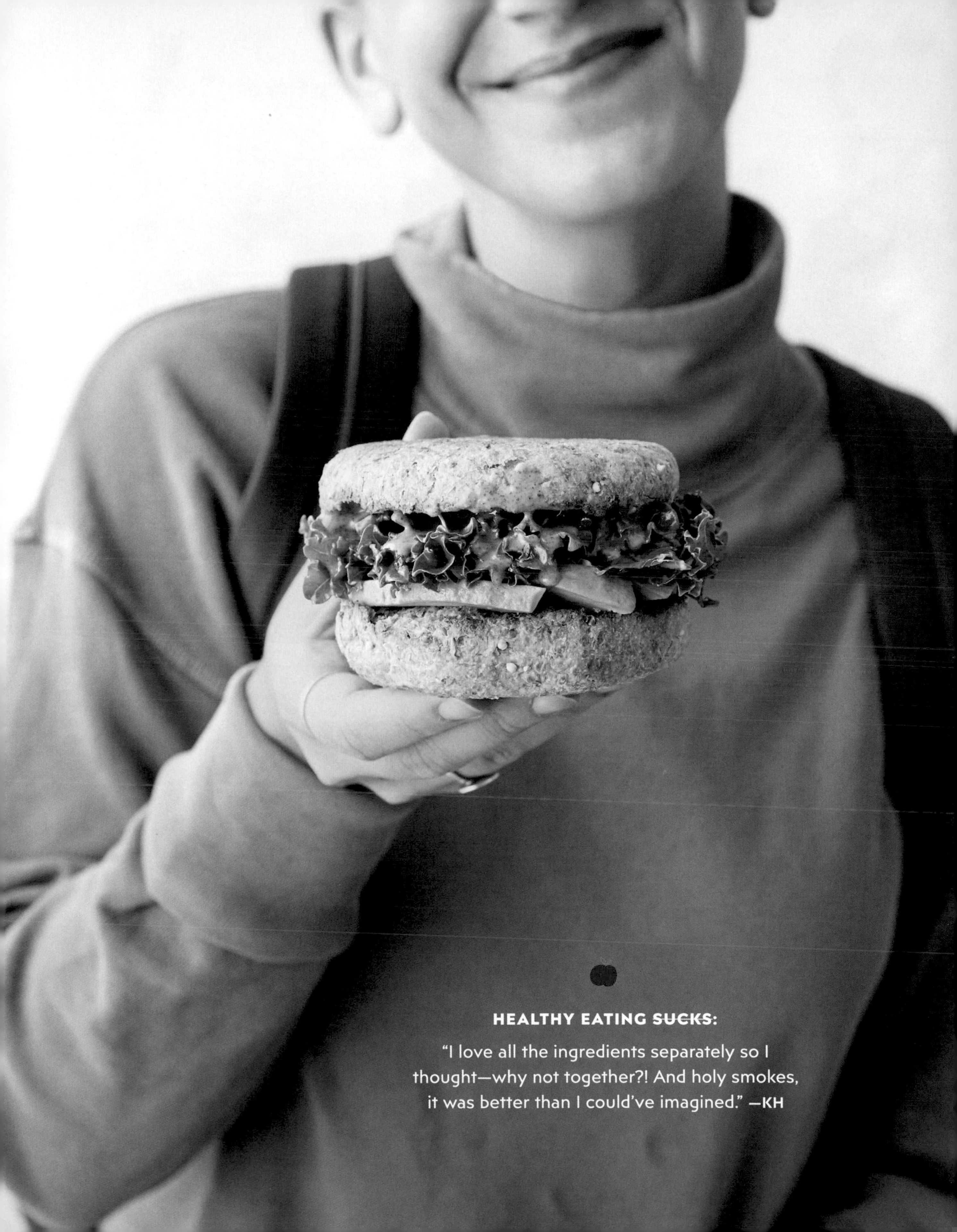

HEALTHY EATING ~~SUCKS~~:

"I love all the ingredients separately so I thought—why not together?! And holy smokes, it was better than I could've imagined." —**KH**

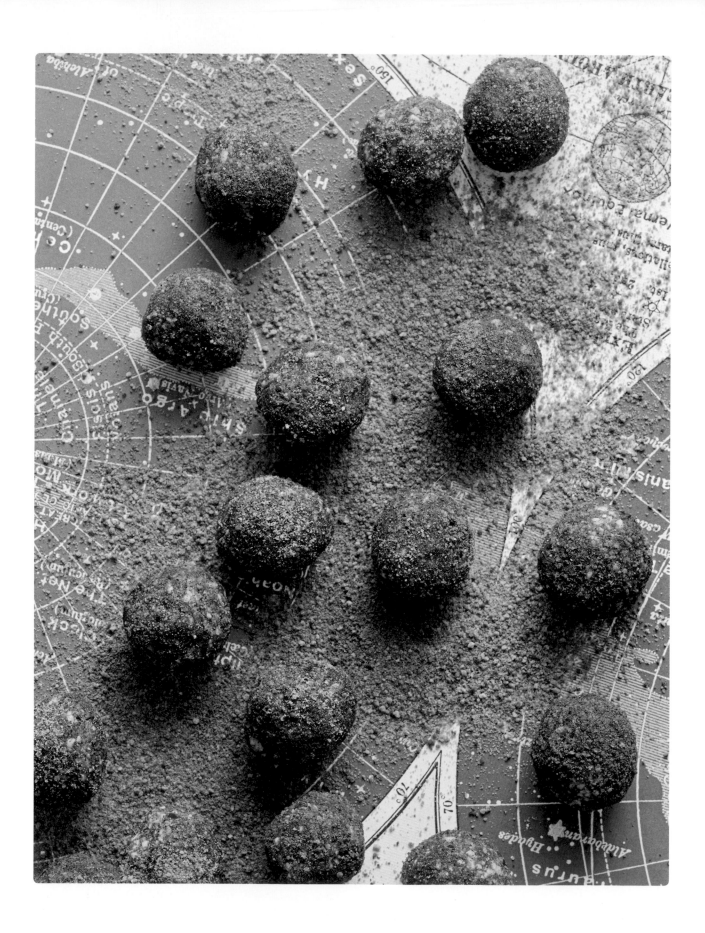

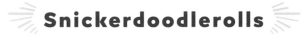

Snickerdoodlerolls

These little guys have been compared to the inner ring of a cinnamon roll, making them satisfying snacks for any situation. Their flyness can help distract you from the fears, frustrations, and freaky parts of hurtling through the sky. If you want extra chill-out mojo, add reishi powder—the Zen-ist mushroom in all the kingdom.

MAKES 20 (FEEL FREE TO HALVE THE RECIPE—BUT WHY WOULD YOU DO THAT?)

1 cup raw cashews

¼ cup vanilla protein powder (oat flour or even rolled oats work, too; if using, process the oats alone first to make them into a flour)

1 packed cup Medjool dates, pitted (16 to 18 dates)

1 teaspoon vanilla extract

2 teaspoons cinnamon

2 tablespoon reishi mushroom powder (optional)

2 tablespoons coconut sugar

1 teaspoon cinnamon

1. In a food processor, pulse the cashews alone until they're the texture of sand. If using rolled oats in place of protein powder, add them now.
2. Add the protein powder, dates, vanilla, cinnamon, 4 teaspoons water, and the mushroom powder, if using, and process until no big chunks remain.
3. In a small bowl, mix the coconut sugar and cinnamon.
4. Roll the batter into little balls; 1 tablespoon per ball = 20 balls.
5. Roll each ball in the cinnamon-sugar mixture.
6. Store in the fridge for max longevity, or in the freezer if it's a hot day.

AFTER [PARTY] THOUGHT:

I keep these in my fridge for emergency snacking, impromptu car trips, "I was gonna eat lunch, but I got a work call so now I have to put something in my body or I'll die" situations, or a late-night treat.

 HEALTHY EATING ~~SUCKS~~:

"Amazing. I have given many to friends and they say it is to die for. I think I have made this recipe eight times and memorized it." **—TM**

WHEN YOU'RE GOING ON A ROAD TRIP, BABY!

Road trips are the easiest to pack for because you usually don't have to limit the amount you bring. My car food tote is larger than the one Reese Witherspoon wore on her back in *Wild* before embarking on an eleven-hundred-mile hike, but at a minimum, I pack an apple, lots of water, and one or both of these snacks.

Curry Car Cashews

Roasted nuts are a classic rest-stop snack, and this oil-free variety packs a level of flavor that, like an uneven one-arm-out-the-car-window tan line, is impossible *not* to comment on.

MAKES 1½ CUPS (DOUBLE OR TRIPLE AS DESIRED)

1½ cups raw cashews

3 tablespoons freshly squeezed lime juice (about 1 really juicy lime)

2 tablespoons curry powder

1 teaspoon sea salt

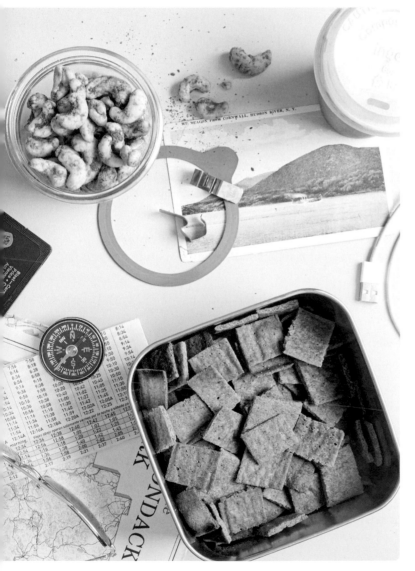

1. Preheat the oven to 250°F. Line a rimmed baking sheet with parchment paper and set aside.
2. Mix the cashews, lime juice, curry powder, and salt in a large bowl, making sure to coat the cashews from head to toe.
3. Spread the cashews on the prepared baking sheet.
4. Bake for 40 minutes, popping into the oven with a spatula to move them around every so often.
5. Remove from the oven and let them cool and get crunchy.
6. Store leftovers in a sealed container on the counter.

AFTER [PARTY] THOUGHT:

My recipe testers adored these curried cuties as an office snack, an instead-of-croutons salad topper, or even a "beer [or kombucha] [or hard apple cider] snack."

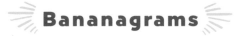

Bananagrams

Not to be confused with the Scrabble-like game by the same name, these Bananagrams are like crunchy bites of banana bread, or sweet graham crackers. Either way, chances are that while you're diving in by the fistful, you'll be unable to think about anything other than *I hope we're not there* [at the bottom of the bag] *yet*.

MAKES A SNACK FOR 2

½ heaping cup mashed ripe banana (about 1 large banana)

¾ cup oat flour

½ teaspoon sea salt or pink salt

2 tablespoons refined coconut oil, melted

½ teaspoon cinnamon

½ teaspoon vanilla extract

2 tablespoons coconut or organic cane/palm sugar

1. Preheat the oven to 350°F. Line a baking sheet with parchment paper.
2. In a large bowl, stir the banana, oat flour, salt, coconut oil, cinnamon, vanilla, and coconut sugar to make a dough.
3. On a baking sheet, use a spatula to spread the dough into a thin, uniform layer.
4. Bake for 10 minutes, then remove from the oven and use a paring knife or pizza cutter to slice into cracker shapes. Flip each cracker with a spatula to bake them evenly.
5. Put them back in the oven for another 10 to 12 minutes, until they're dry and crispy and lightly golden brown.
6. Let the crackers cool and harden up a little more and then dive in.
7. Store leftovers in a sealed container at room temperature for up to 5 days.

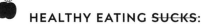 **HEALTHY EATING ~~SUCKS~~:**

"My roommate swore she wouldn't like them and then I caught her sneaking them off the baking tray." **—KB**

NOTE: I tested the bejeezus out of this recipe to make sure that I had exhausted all possible flavor combinations. Make 'em chocolatey by adding 1 tablespoon of cacao powder (with an additional sprinkle of chocolate chips/cacao nibs on top before baking), or peanut buttery by adding 2 tablespoons of peanut butter (with an additional sprinkle of coconut flakes).

WHEN YOU'RE A GUEST IN SOMEONE'S HOME

Going with the flow can mess with your flow, sanity—and digestion. And that can make you an unpleasant, ungrateful, and unhappy houseguest. When you're staying in someone's home, practice putting on your own oxygen mask first. Self-caring is the best way to be your best self—and get the most repeat invites.

You can't just hijack someone else's kitchen and dictate all the meals, but you *can* take over your plate by bringing your own condiments to improve the quality of your food. By condiments, I mean easily packable and nonperishable goods like:

- stevia for calorie-free, sugar-less sweetness in oatmeal, tea, coffee, cocktails

- apple cider vinegar to add to your water to boost digestion, hydration, energy, and metabolism

- plant-protein powders to make protein pancakes and stir into yogurt

- tea—which is a choice way to take care of yourself in a nonintrusive way. (See page 265 for ideas.)

- chia seeds for yogurts, peanut butter toasts, oatmeal, even ice cream, and to make chia puddings.

- popcorn (page 224)

Beyond packing these condiments in with my socks, I've found sneaky success disguising foods for myself as gifts for my host. Gift homemade treats that you also want to eat! These two recipes are my "thanks for having me, don't mind if I do" go-to's:

Very Present-able Pecans

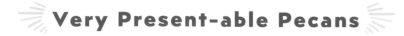

These sweet and salty roasted pecans aren't only an appropriate gift for your host but a gift for your mouth, too. Whether it's a housewarming, holiday party, or an engagement brunch, the reactions I've received upon gifting these nuts makes me feel nuts to ever gift anything from Amazon again.

MAKES SLIGHTLY MORE THAN ONE 16-OUNCE BALL JAR FULL

2 cups raw pecans (try to find whole or halves, not pieces)

1½ tablespoons maple syrup

½ teaspoon cinnamon

¼ teaspoon sea salt or pink salt

1. Preheat the oven to 375°F. Line a rimmed baking sheet with parchment paper.
2. In a large bowl, combine the pecans with the maple syrup, cinnamon, and salt. Stir well to cover all of the pecans evenly.
3. Spread the pecans on the baking sheet and slide it into the oven.
4. Bake for 10 minutes; swoop into the oven halfway through to move the pecans around so they cook evenly.
5. Remove from the oven and let them cool for at least 20 minutes—they'll harden up.
6. Gift in a glass ball jar with a ribbon decoration if you're good at that kind of thing (I wish I was).

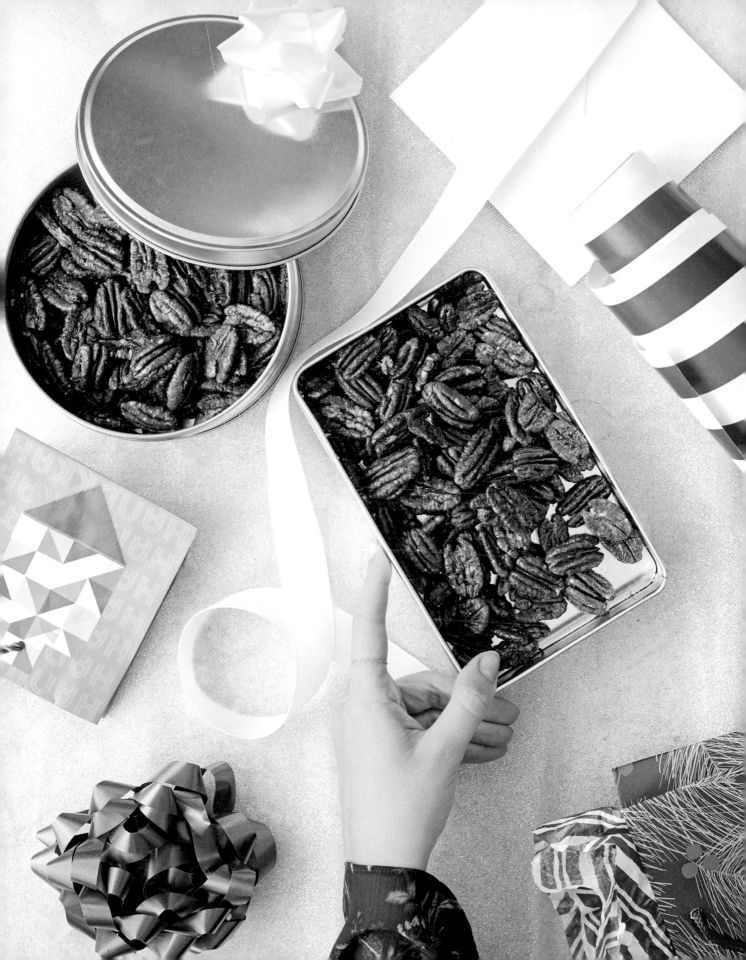

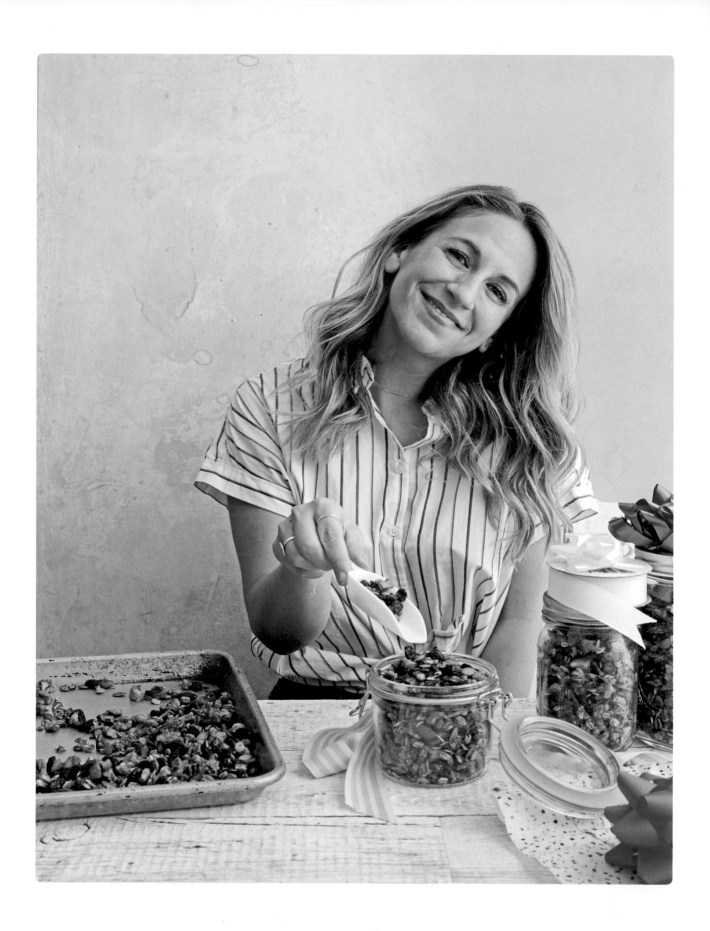

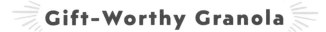

Gift-Worthy Granola

If I turned my apartment into an Airbnb—or operated an actual B&B—I would leave a jar of this citrus cranberry granola for every guest, and even if I never scrubbed the shower or made the bed, I'd be guaranteed five-star status. That's just how good it is. If you don't believe me, ask my dad. Every time I go visit my parents, he shamelessly begs me to bring a jar.

MAKES ABOUT 10 CUPS (SAID DIFFERENTLY: A LOT)

1½ cups old-fashioned rolled oats (not the quick-cooking kind) (gluten-free if you need them to be)

3 cups raw pecans, almonds, or walnuts (or a combo), chopped or food processed into whatever size nut chunks you like your granola to have (you can put your nuts in the food processor to chop to make your life easier!)

1 tablespoon lemon zest (I hate zesting, too, but it's worth it)

1 tablespoon orange zest

2 tablespoons freshly squeezed orange juice

¾ teaspoon sea salt

2 teaspoons cinnamon

2 teaspoons vanilla extract

½ cup maple syrup

1 cup raw pumpkin seeds (pepitas)

1 cup raisins

1 cup dried cranberries

¼ cup plain unsweetened applesauce

1 large apple of any kind you love, coarsely chopped

1. Preheat the oven to 325°F.

2. In a large mixing bowl, mix the oats, nuts, lemon zest, orange zest, orange juice, salt, cinnamon, vanilla, maple syrup, pumpkin seeds, if using, raisins, cranberries, applesauce, and apple together.

3. Spread the granola mixture right onto a rimmed baking sheet (no need for parchment).

4. Bake for 20 minutes, then pop into the oven and mix around so it cooks evenly.

5. Bake for another 25 to 35 minutes or until it looks golden brown. It'll harden up once you remove it, so don't panic if it's golden but not crunchy.

6. Remove from the oven and let it cool, then enjoy the party in your mouth! Or in almond milk or yogurt. Or package up in a pretty glass jar as a gift to someone else's lucky mouth.

7. Store leftovers at room temperature in a sealed container.

AFTER [PARTY] THOUGHT:

You know that store-bought granola is one of the biggest scams out there, right? Maybe because outdoorsy folks originally put granola on the map, it got a healthy rep, but really, it's the Fyre Fest of snacks since it's typically full of crappy oils, sugar, and low-quality grains. Don't be intimidated by making your own; this is one of the easiest recipes in this entire book.

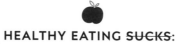

HEALTHY EATING ~~SUCKS~~:

"Wow, I am never buying my own granola again. I loved it and am excited that it'll store super easy too!" —MD

HEALTHY EATING IN THE OFFICE

You can't have your office PLANt Party without a PLAN. Thrive in the place where you spend your 9:00 to 5:00 by stocking your desk drawers with more than Witeout (which I thought was extinct until I hand-wrote all of my wedding thank-you notes and went through a whole bottle). Here's what to keep in your desk so feeling good doesn't feel like work:

- Raw or dry roasted nuts

- Popcorn (BYO or find a kind that comes in coconut oil, not butter)

- Nut butter (for spreading on fresh fruit, rice crackers, or celery)

- Fresh fruit (the semi-nonperishable kinds like bananas, apples, oranges, and grapefruit)

- Rice crackers

- Celery (and/or carrot sticks, sliced bell peppers, even raw snap peas)

- Dark chocolate

- Dried fruit (dates, goji berries, crystalized ginger, mango, peach, etc.)

- Chia seeds

- Protein powder

- Greens powder

- Emergency exit bars

- Tea bags*

- Bananagrams (page 258), Cheeseisn'ts (page 88), Curry Car Cashews (page 257), Gift-Worthy Granola (page 263), Cacao Crumbs (page 316)

Pop these into your office fridge:

- Coconut water
- Fruit (the perishable kinds like berries, pineapple, and mango)
- Hummus
- Kombucha
- Nondairy yogurt
- Smoothies

---

*There's a T for Every Y   ᶻᶻᶻᶻ

I want to spill some tea about tea. Whatever ailment you've got, there is an infusion to help make things better.

You're Low on Energy

Green tea and yerba maté are your best friends when you need an energizing boost. Yerba maté, in particular, is wonderful because it won't make you jittery and is high in metabolism-boosting nutrients and antioxidants. (It was called "the drink of the gods" by indigenous South Americans, so I mean, why wouldn't you want it?)

You Can't Fall Asleep

When you can't fall asleep, there's nothing like chamomile or magnesium (and a boring book) to save you. Chamomile has mild sedative effects, which help knock you out, and magnesium relaxes your nervous system, which helps you sleep more soundly through the night.

You Feel Bloated

When bloat is your woe, drink dandelion. It's a liver cleanser, which means it helps the liver function and encourages the production of bile, regulating the digestive system (a.k.a. getting stuff out the other end). Dandelion tea is also a natural diuretic, which makes it the perfect tea to relieve bloating and water retention.

Your Digestion Needs a Leg Up

Ginger is the goddess of good digestion. It can calm a regular upset stomach and even curb nausea. In India, it is known as the "universal medicine," because in addition to helping alleviate gas and bloating, helping us "go," and

ᶻᶻᶻᶻ

soothing our tummies, ginger's also great at helping our bodies heat up from the inside—a plus on any cold day.

You're Stressed or Cranky

Lemon balm lifts your spirits. Make sure you stop and smell the tea leaves because it's been used for centuries in aromatherapy, too; the sweet aroma of its oil can encourage feelings of relaxation and calm.

You Gotta, Um, Eliminate

Senna leaf is your jam when you're jammed up. It stimulates intestinal contractions (helping wake up your colon to get things moving), and increases fluids and electrolytes in the colon. (This is all a fancy way of saying it's a laxative.) Buyer beware: Drink this when you know you'll have a good twelve hours at home to enjoy the effects.

You're Feeling Under the Weather

It's not technically a tea, but you can't go wrong by squeezing fresh lemon juice into hot water. High in vitamin C, which is stellar for fighting colds, lemon water is a superstar for our immunity. It also helps balance our pH (alkalize our bodies), which kicks acid-thriving diseases to the curb.

WHEN YOU HAVE TO EAT ON YOUR COMMUTE

Texting while driving is a big hell no, and so is skipping breakfast. When brekky must take place from the driver's seat (or while waiting for the subway), you gotta do what you gotta do. And just like texting and driving don't mix, spoons and steering wheels don't, either. They say, "Let the message wait . . . control your fate," and I say, "Eat these protein-packed muffins that taste like cookie dough while you drive to the place where you earn your spending dough." HEYO!

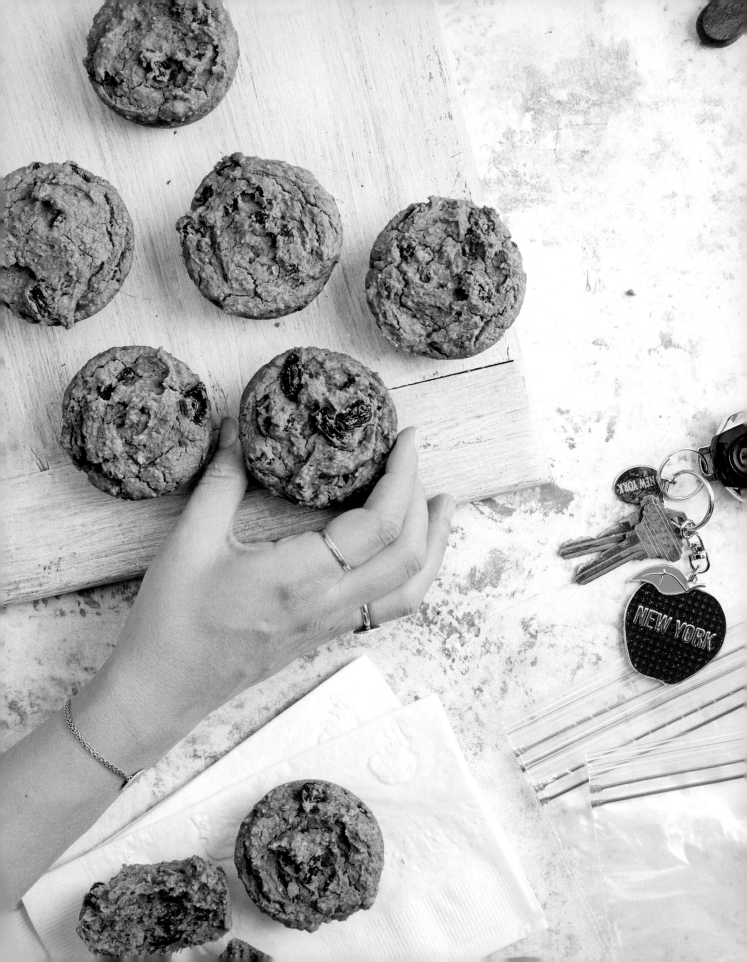

Chickpea Protein Muffins

1 15-ounce can chickpeas, drained, rinsed, and shaken dry

½ cup almond butter

¼ cup maple syrup

½ teaspoon cinnamon

2 teaspoons vanilla extract

¼ teaspoon salt

¼ teaspoon baking powder

¼ teaspoon baking soda

2 tablespoons rolled oats

Raisins, chocolate chips, fresh or frozen berries, or dried cranberries with shaved orange peel (optional)

Coconut oil spray, to grease the muffin tin

1. Preheat the oven to 350°F. Spray a muffin tin with coconut oil spray.
2. Place the chickpeas, almond butter, maple syrup, cinnamon, vanilla, salt, baking powder, baking soda, and oats in a food processor or blender and process them together. The batter will be thick.
3. Stir in the raisins or other treats if using.
4. Spoon the batter into the muffin cups.
5. Bake for 20 to 25 minutes for regular-size muffins. (Cooking time will vary with mini-muffins.) They're done when they look golden, even though they might be a little mushy. If you let them cook too long, they'll become crumbly.
6. Let cool before diving in.
7. Store in a sealed container in the fridge and eat leftovers out of the fridge or reheated in the toaster oven or microwave.

AFTER [PARTY] THOUGHT:

Nix the baking part and keep the batter as a tasty dip for apple slices or on a spoon. (That's why this recipe doubles as a cookie dough for when you need to eat your feelings on page 132.)

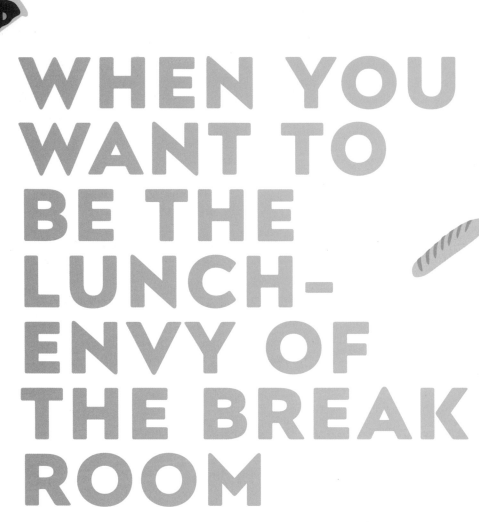

WHEN YOU WANT TO BE THE LUNCH-ENVY OF THE BREAK ROOM

#LEFTOVERSARETHEBESTOVERS has never been more true than when it comes to work lunch. It's like "Command + C"ing last night's food and "Command + V"ing it today. If you don't have a full leftover lunch from a prior meal, then gather up your scraps and build a wrap.

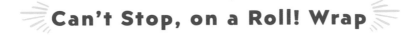

Can't Stop, on a Roll! Wrap

I am that obnoxious person who forgets to eat lunch. I chalk it up to being so engulfed in what I do and doing it by myself—it's not like I get social cues from my three-hole punch that it's chow time. So when it finally hits me that I was due to eat T-minus 2 hours ago, I need something quick that won't interrupt my flow. That's where this lunch came from. All you do is grab every rogue plant scrap that you saved or stocked, throw them in a wrap smeared with Tahini Miso Magic Sauce (page 273), and bring this hodgepodge to flava town.

SERVES 1

Plant protein you have lying around
(a can of beans, thawed frozen
edamame, a veggie burger, leftover
tofu or tempeh)

Rogue veggies from your fridge
(handful of spinach or kale,
½ bell pepper, shredded carrots,
⅓ cucumber)

½ cup refrigerated premade quinoa

Handful of sprouts

1 leftover spread or sauce of choice
(Red Peppa Pesto on page 209,
Besto Pesto on page 200, Crazy-
Quick Fettuccine Caulifredo
Spaghetti Squasho on page 121), but
the best is Tahini Miso Magic Sauce
(page 273)

1 large tortilla (brown rice, sprouted
grain, spelt, a collard green,
whatever you like)

1. Consolidate the protein, veggies, quinoa, sprouts, and spread a wrap.
2. Eat.

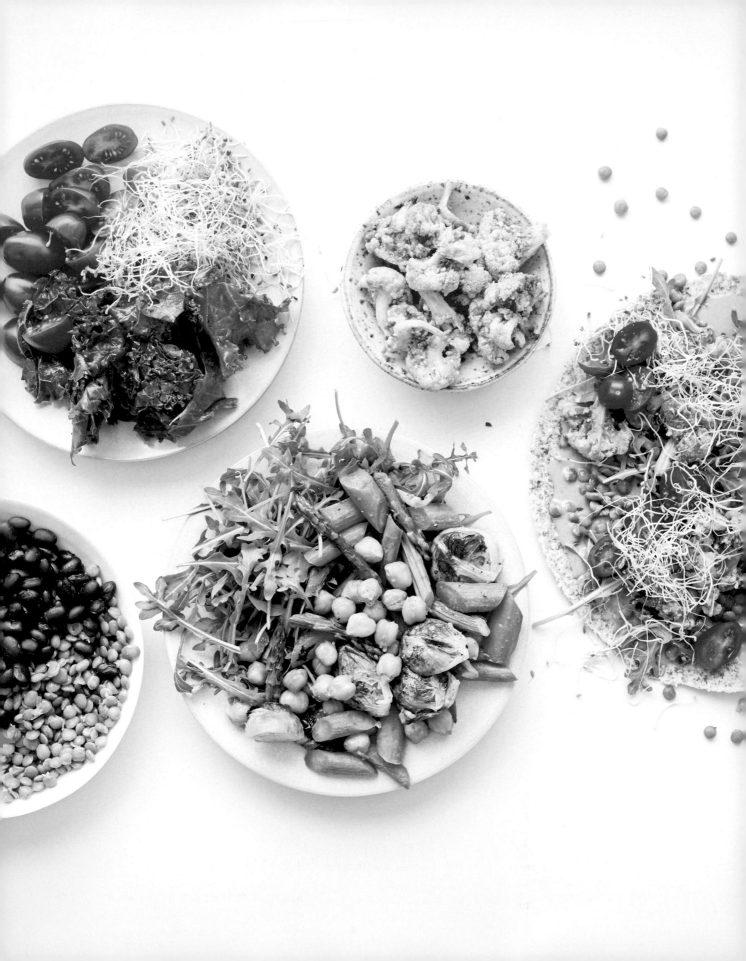

TAHINI MISO MAGIC SAUCE

After spending thirty seconds and three ingredients making this tahini miso sauce, *it* spends its next moments of life transforming leftovers into bestovers. It works as a spread for wraps, sandwiches, and toasts; it adds moisture to leftover grains, beans, sweet potatoes, and pasta; and it'll quickly dress any salad. It's amazing as a shampoo, too. Okay, no, just kidding. But not kidding that having this sauce up your sleeve will make eating healthier magically easier.

MAKES ABOUT 3 SERVINGS

¼ cup tahini

2 tablespoon miso (I love the "sweet white miso" variety)

3 tablespoon apple cider vinegar

1. In a bowl, jar, or glass measuring cup, add the tahini, miso, vinegar, and 1 tablespoon water. Use a fork to stir to combine really well.

2. Add more water to make it more like a dressing, or leave it thick for a spread texture.

3. Store leftovers in a sealed container in the fridge.

WHEN YOU'VE JUST STRAIGHT-UP CRASHED AT 3:00

The afternoon slump may be a cliché, but much like a baby boomer not knowing how to use Facebook, it's all too true. (As proven by my dad wishing my mom a happy birthday on his own wall. And then replying to his own post.) Rather than fight the inevitable, I rely on matcha, which you already met on page 3, to help me get the job done.

Matcha Mint Chocolate Chip Energy Balls

Listen, we can point fingers at our desperate desire to catch z's in between emails or our circadian rhythms or a post-lunch blood-sugar drop, or we can bypass blame and make these to have on hand for p.m. crash-rehabilitation.

MAKES 12 BALLS

½ packed cup Medjool dates (7 or 8 dates), pitted

¼ cup rolled oats (not the quick-cooking kind)

2½ tablespoons almond butter

1 to 2 teaspoons matcha

2 tablespoons chocolate plant-protein powder (I use Chocolate Sunwarrior Classic Protein)

¼ cup tightly packed fresh mint leaves, washed and dried

2 tablespoons chocolate chips

1. Place the dates, oats, almond butter, matcha, protein powder, and mint in a food processor and process until it looks like coarse sand.

2. If it looks dry, add water, 1 teaspoon at a time, until it looks a bit moister and stickier.

3. Add the chocolate chips and pulse to break them into whatever size chunks tickle your fancy.

4. Get in there and roll your dough into balls, baby. 1 tablespoon per ball = 12 balls.

5. Store in an airtight container in your fridge for up to 2 weeks.

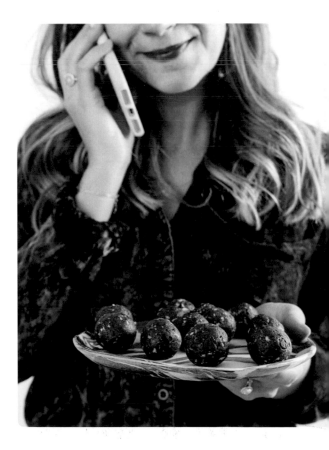

☽ AFTER [PARTY] THOUGHT:

Not everyone loves the taste of matcha, so these recipes are more about its energy-boosting powers, but up the matcha if you'd like a stronger flavor.

Mix-and-Match-a Matcha Latte

Similar to the whole "save a horse, ride a cowboy" embargo, this is my "save a silly matcha latte frother, use a blender" homemade matcha latte recipe. Four years ago, I bought my husband a matcha latte frother and it was a bigger waste than when I bought that head scratcher from Sharper Image. Trust me: Ride your blender off into the matcha latte sunset.

SERVES 1 (DOUBLE OR TRIPLE AS DESIRED)

1 cup plain, unsweetened almond milk (or any other plant milk)

1 teaspoon matcha

Natural sweetener to taste, such as stevia; ½ teaspoon coconut sugar; 1 Medjool date; or 1 teaspoon organic cane sugar, palm sugar, honey, or maple syrup

A bonus: collagen peptides, MCT oil, CBD oil, coconut butter

1. Pulse the almond milk, matcha, sweetener, and bonus ingredients, if using, together in a blender.

2. For iced: Pour over ice and drink.

3. For hot: Transfer the contents from the blender to a small saucepan and heat to your desired temperature. I like to bring it to a light boil and then immediately turn off the heat and pour it into a mug.

AFTER [PARTY] THOUGHT:

Add a splash of vanilla extract, ¼ to ½ teaspoon cinnamon, maca, pumpkin pie spice, ground ginger, or even some chai tea to bring this matcha to flava town.

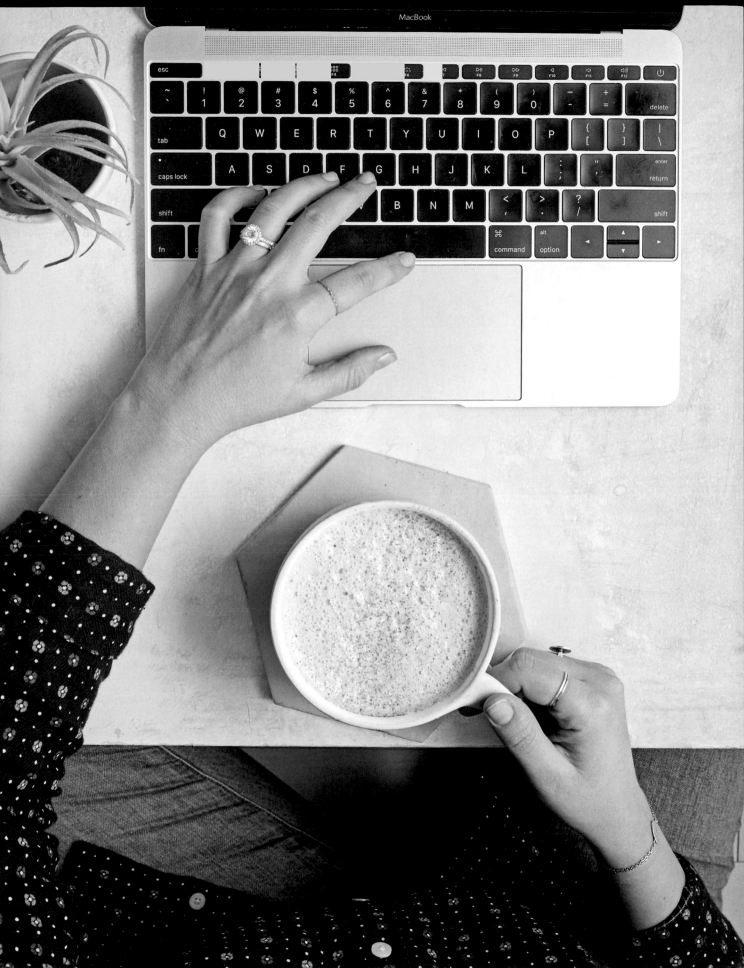

WHEN YOU HAVE AN OFFICE PARTY, BUT YOU DON'T WANT TO PISS OFF THE PLANNING COMMITTEE

Full disclosure: My main experience with office life has been watching *The Office*. Like eight times through, though. Which is enough to learn that office parties are a big deal, happen often and for random occasions, and involve peer pressure to eat the celebratory crap. That said, bringing Fooled Ya Black Bean Brownies (page 279) is more exciting than when you got a desk chair with lumbar support. And much like that desk chair, you can lean on this recipe for every occasion from Claire from Accounting's baby shower, Joe from IT's birthday party, *and* the Secret Santa reveal.

Fooled Ya Black Bean Brownies

What's with the "fooled ya" thing? These brownies are as much a trick as they are a treat. They fool the taste buds into thinking that they're an unhealthy, diet-ruining, guilt-provoking dessert, but really, they're an uber healthy, diet-friendly, smile-provoking treat made from freaking beans. So unlike when Jim pranks Dwight, this is one prank that will please everyone.

MAKES ONE 8 X 8-INCH OR 9 X 9-INCH PAN, 9 AVERAGE-SIZE BROWNIES OR 18 BROWNIE BITES

1 15-ounce can black beans, drained and rinsed

⅔ cup almond butter or peanut butter

2 tablespoons cocoa powder or cacao powder

½ cup coconut sugar, organic sugar, or raw cane sugar

1 teaspoon baking powder

½ to 1 cup chocolate chips

Coconut oil spray, for greasing the pan (optional)

1. Preheat the oven to 350°F. Line an 8 x 8-inch or 9 x 9-inch baking pan with parchment paper or spray it with coconut oil, if using.
2. Place the beans, almond butter, cocoa powder, coconut sugar, and baking powder in a food processor and process it up. After about a minute, use a spatula to scrape down the sides, then process again until smooth.
3. Remove the blade from the food processor and set it aside. Do *not* lick the blade, as tempting as it will be.
4. Add the chocolate chips to the bowl of the food processor and use a spatula to mix them in so they're evenly distributed.
5. Add the batter to the prepared pan. Use a spatula to spread it out so it's evenly distributed.
6. Bake for 20 to 25 minutes. Touch the top of the brownies; they're ready when they bounce back up quickly. Or consider them done if a toothpick slides out clean.
7. Let them cool for at least 10 minutes. Cut them into whatever sizes you'd like.
8. Don't forget to hide any sign of the mystery ingredient until everyone's devoured them and is asking, "OMG what are *in* these?!"

NOTE: Some smarty-pants recipe testers baked these into cookies using a cookie scoop and a baking sheet and said they baked even quicker this way.

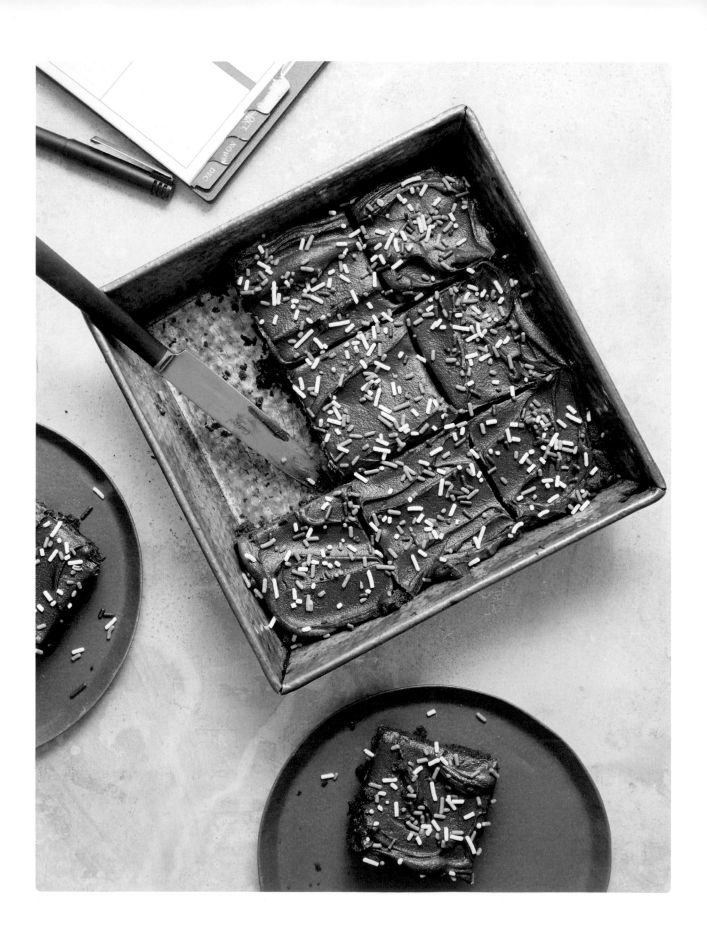

AFTER [PARTY] THOUGHT:

The enjoyment of these brownies is not limited to places with copy machines. They're a special treat for any party, and they pack up perfectly in a picnic basket or lunch box. They're also a cure for any chocolate craving and anytime you get dumped.

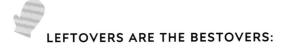

LEFTOVERS ARE THE BESTOVERS:

Store in a sealed container or wrapped up in the fridge and consider enjoying them chopped in a bowl of Banana Ice Cream (page 110).

HEALTHY EATING ~~SUCKS~~:

"My boyfriend was so hesitant to even give them a shot, but he took a bite of the batter and then was literally begging for one when they came out of the oven. Not sure we'll ever be able to go back to normal brownies." **—MC**

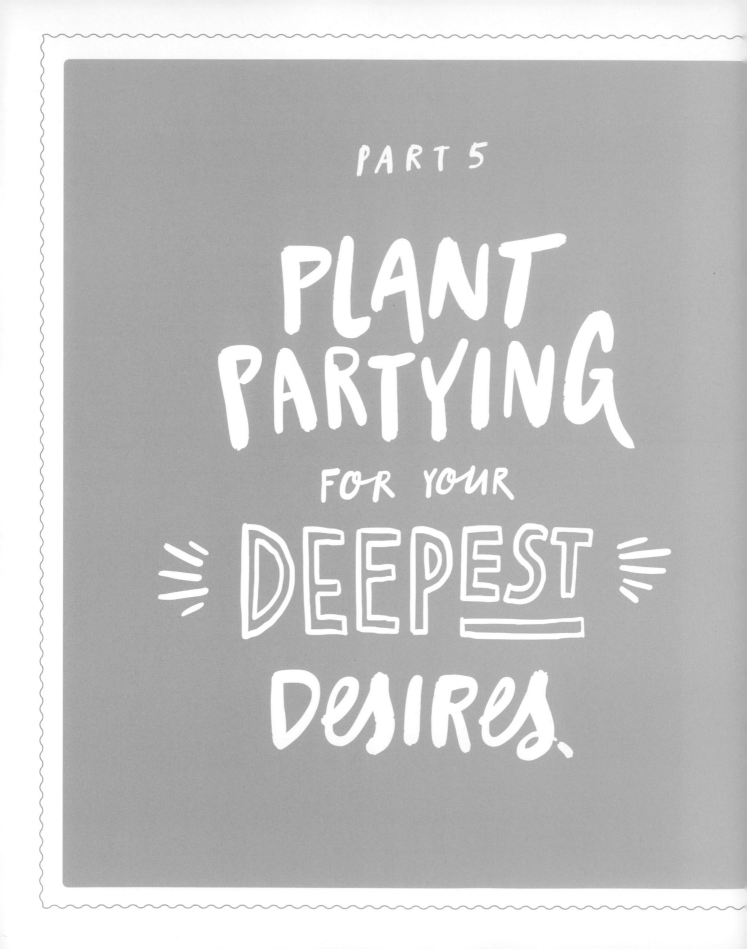

PART 5

PLANT PARTYING

FOR YOUR

=DEEPEST=

Desires.

(or just your cravings)

Sorry it's taken me 282 pages to spill the pinto beans that a *Party in Your Plants* diet can help you find a happy, comfortable weight—it doesn't really count as a weight-loss diet. But you knew that, right?

"Healthy eating" isn't the new Atkins, Zone, South Beach, North Beach, Laguna Beach, topless beach, whatever diet. Healthy eating is the only real route to feeling, looking, thinking, and living your best. This is something that I hear from women I coach or share sangria with: "I eat well, but I can't lose weight. What's the point?" I sigh and use my peaceful yogi voice to explain that eating well doesn't always mean eating for weight loss. The calories in organic almond butter are still calories. Just because something's healthy doesn't mean you can eat unlimited amounts and expect it not to affect your waistline.

Your body doesn't get a memo that the cookies you're eating while emotionally watching *This Is Us* are gluten-free and give them a free pass. Not to throw my sister under the bus—sorry, Nina, I love you, but come on, girlfriend. Not that long ago, she rolled into my apartment munching on a scone while telling me how she was trying to slim down. I asked her what the dealio was with that and she said, "It's healthy! It's made with quinoa!" It's all good; I just want to remind you that healthy and skinny are not the dancing emoji twin girls.

What to Count Instead of Calories

I've never been a calorie counter. Partly because my brain doesn't seem to relate well to numbers and also because my gut knows that it's a bigger waste of time than folding undies. In high school, I tried Weight Watchers and gave up the moment I couldn't tell whether my slice of bread was considered "medium" or "large." (I will say that Weight Watchers did get something right when they made fresh fruits and veggies equal zero points, practically bribing people to eat them.)

So counting might not fall within my definition of a healthy diet, but "checking" definitely is. When you get into your car, you adjust your seat, click your seat belt, tweak your mirrors, and make sure your foot is on the brake before stepping on the gas. Likewise, I do a little checkadoodledo of three important things before I eat.

> Plants—Is there at least one plant on my plate? Ideally, is half my plate plants? Perfectly, is *more* than half of my plate plants?

> Colors—Are the plants different colors? Matching neutrals might be cool at J.Crew but not to nourish you. Is there something green among any orange or tan stuff?

> Blessings—Am I in a chill state of mind? Am I watching the horrible news or reading stressful emails or fighting with a telemarketer because apparently those are a thing again? Is my nervous system feeling relaxed? Even better, am I feeling appreciation for this colorful meal I'm about to dive fork first into?

BONUS THING TO COUNT: CHEWS

It's not just passionate moments with your lover that begin with our mouths, it's where digestion begins, too! Our teeth and digestive enzymes in our saliva start the breaking-down process. Chewing more means we're more likely to notice when we're full, and it can reduce digestive distress and help us reap the most benefits of whatever we're eating so the vitamins and minerals don't just go from tongue to toilet without seeping into our systems. (Hello, whole peas in our poo!)

Try chewing a mouthful about fifteen times and see if it doesn't slow down your eating, encourage you to eat more mindfully, and lessen digestive distress and, bonus: help you stay more mindful when you eat.

JUST EAT A LIIIIITLE LESS

I live in New York City, where eating out at one of its twenty-four thousand restaurants (and that's in Manhattan alone) is a way of life. Although it's easy enough to seek out spots that prioritize organic produce and good-quality oils, sweeteners, and salts, when I'm sipping wine over a flickering candle across from my honey, it's not always easy to decide what to get. So we often order three dishes. Or four. (One time we did seven, but I don't want to talk about it.)

What this does, besides eliciting many audible MMMM's and circular tummy rubs, is stretch my midriff muscle. Our stomachs are like a muscle, by the way! The distensibility (the supersmart term for the amount our stomach walls can stretch) increases and decreases—just like our glutes.

When I was a few months away from my wedding, I found myself stereotypically engulfed in way too many not-important-in-hindsight high-emotion discussions with my now husband (yay, we made it) over dinner. Since I know we feel crummy when we eat even good food with bad vibes, I found myself taking much smaller portions. Soon, I just needed less food than I had needed before to feel full. Thanks distensibility decrease! It was sweet because I looked banging in my dress without consciously restricting myself. I just ate a little less.

PRIORITIZE PLANT PROTEIN

Focus on getting plant protein in every meal or snack. Whatever your goal—weight loss, sustained energy, a balanced mood, hitting the gym more—that's the golden ticket. It'll help you fill up faster, eat less, feel stronger, recover from workouts quicker, think sharper, fight off colds easier, balance your blood sugar better, and keep your waistline slimmer.

Many of my clients don't even know where to begin. They tell me, "I eat lots of nut butter," which rocks. But nut butter isn't the only source of plant protein out there, my friends. (And it's not even a welcome source because it's hard to digest due to its high fat content, which we'll get into in a moment.) Better? Lentils, black beans, chickpeas, oats, hemp seeds, chia seeds, quinoa, tempeh, tofu (non-GMO, organic), edamame, and plant-protein powder.

DON'T GO NUTS ON NUTS

We're living in a time when pounds of peanut, almond, and sunflower butter get dumped by the cupful into food bloggers' oatmeal and smoothie bowls. I've had dozens of clients come to me feeling pumped because they're eating so much almond butter, and that's healthy, right? Sure. It's not *unhealthy*. Nuts are nutritious, their fat is A++ for our bods, they provide some protein and fiber, they balance our blood sugar and make us less hungry after eating. But we're talking a tablespoon. *Maybe* two. Have you ever portioned out a tablespoon of nut butter? It's depressing. Your bread would barely be buttered, and for roughly 100 calories (the equivalent of six almonds).

Let me back up. I said that I don't count calories. I don't even eat food that comes with calorie labels. But I've come to understand that even the healthiest of fat can be *a lot* to digest. When we use buckets of nut butter on our oatmeal, toasts, smoothie bowls, sweet potatoes, bananas, spoons, and fingers, it adds up big time.

EAT. MORE. PLANTS.

The antidote to eating lots of gooey processed nuts is eating real, fresh fruits and vegetables. It's pretty impossible to consume too much kale, or to eat your weight in apples. Let's get back to the definition of Partying in Your Plants—"eating more plants than you do crap," with "crap" being: chemicals, refined, artificial, and processed foods. This is the ultimate weight-loss plan: Eat fewer foods with portion sizes written on their labels, because if there's a label there's a good chance it's full of CRAP, and eat more foods like bell peppers and pears, which have no labels nor limits. These infinite-possibility fruits, veggies, and legumes also have a ton of fiber, which fills you up and requires you to eat less to be good to go.

WHEN YOU WANNA GUARANTEE THAT YOUR FAVORITE DRESS WILL STILL ZIP

I thought I was pretty cool when, at age twenty-six, I wore my senior prom dress to our friends' black-tie wedding. Now I realize that it was silly to wear an outdated teenybopper dress to an adult affair, but I'm still pretty proud I was able to do it. That's the thing with eating plants; it helps you stay at your natural weight with ease. And here's the thing about these strategic slimming recipes that follow: eating them in place of higher-calorie meals a couple of times a week starting two weeks before a high-pressure event will ensure that no seams bust while you're doing the cha-cha slide.

LEFTOVERS ARE THE BESTOVERS:

Besides eating chia pudding by way of a spoon, consider eating chia
pudding by way of topping protein pancakes with the pudding or mixing it
into Banana Ice Cream (page 110).

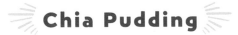

Chia Pudding

When you want to get into bikini (or trunks) shape pronto, there's no doubt that eating slightly less than normal and exercising slightly more than normal will work in your favor. But one thing that doesn't work in your favor is eating flavorless low-calorie food. This chia pudding is what I make to trick my taste buds into thinking I'm chowing down on something decadent, without my love handles agreeing. Because chia seeds are high in fiber and protein, this will fill you up, and because it's an energizing treat, you'll have more gusto to get your dance on.

SERVES 1

3 tablespoons chia seeds

1 cup almond milk or other plant milk

1 to 3 teaspoons honey or maple syrup or a few drops/sprinkles of stevia

1. Mix the chia seeds, almond milk, and honey together in a jar. An empty nut butter or sauce jar works just fine.
2. Pop it into the fridge. Get in there after 3 to 5 minutes and stir to make sure the chia seeds are well mixed throughout.
3. Put it back into the fridge for at least 20 to 30 minutes, even overnight.
4. Top with fruits, seeds, and spices of your choice.

A different chia for every dia

Coffee Cacao (Substitute ½ cup coffee, chilled, plus ½ cup almond milk and top with 1 tablespoon cacao nibs.)

Matcha (Blend ½ teaspoon matcha into the almond milk before stirring in the chia seeds.)

Orange Zest (Mix in ½ teaspoon orange zest plus ⅛ to ¼ teaspoon vanilla extract plus top with 1 tablespoon chopped raw walnuts.)

Chocolate Strawberry (Blend 2 tablespoons cocoa powder or cacao powder plus a pinch of sea salt into the almond milk before stirring in the chia seeds. Top with cacao nibs or chopped strawberries.)

PB & Banana (Stir in 1 to 2 tablespoons peanut butter plus top with ½ banana, sliced, and a pinch of cinnamon.)

Tropical (Stir in 1 to 2 tablespoons coconut flakes plus top with ½ cup chopped mango or pineapple.)

Chai Apple Pie (Blend ½ teaspoon cinnamon, ¼ teaspoon cloves, ¼ teaspoon allspice, and a pinch of nutmeg into the almond milk before stirring in the chia seeds; top with chopped apple.)

Zoodles Plantanesca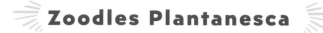

You know how at one point, gym clothes and all other places clothes used to be separate concepts? Well, once upon a time, so did flavorful food and low-calorie food (and vegan food, too). This dish is the athleisure wear of recipes, combining mind-blowing taste with a low calorie count to create something that'll feel as good as wearing yoga pants to happy hour.

SERVES 4

½ to 1 cup cooked green lentils*

1 28-ounce can chunky tomato sauce, regular tomato sauce, or crushed tomatoes in juices or diced tomatoes in juices

½ cup olives, coarsely chopped, plus 1 tablespoon olive juice

1 2-ounce jar capers (about ⅓ cup) plus 1 tablespoon caper juice

3 garlic cloves, finely chopped

1 cup spinach, finely chopped

¼ teaspoon sea salt or pink salt

½ teaspoon crushed red pepper flakes

4 zucchini (1 zucchini per person)

Olive oil, for cooking the zoodles (optional)

¼ to ½ cup fresh parsley (or even more if you're obsessed)

1. * Add ½ cup green lentils to a small saucepan with 1 cup of water and bring to a boil/aggressive simmer, then reduce the heat to a light simmer for 15 to 20 minutes or until the water is absorbed.

2. In a medium saucepan over medium-high heat, combine the tomato sauce, olives and olive juice, capers and caper juice, garlic, spinach, salt, and red pepper flakes. Add the lentils. Bring everything to a simmer, then reduce the heat to a low simmer for about 20 minutes. Stir often until it's not super saucy.

3. Spiralize your zucchinis into zoodles.

4. If you like to cook your zoodles (versus eating them raw), sauté them in a pan over medium heat with a splash of olive oil until soft.

continued

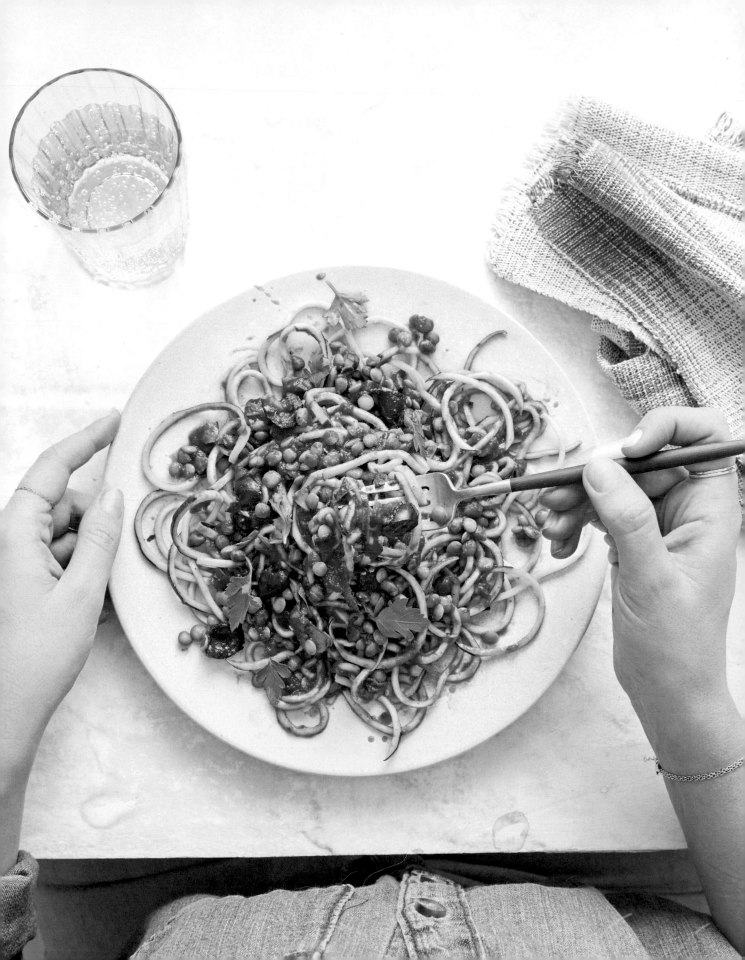

5. Turn off the heat and stir in the chopped parsley.

6. Slather the sauce over your zoodles and stir to combine. Top each serving with an additional sprinkle of fresh parsley.

7. Store leftover sauce in a sealed container in the fridge.

LEFTOVERS ARE THE BESTOVERS:

Leftover sauce but no more zoodles? Try it over quinoa.

Slim-Down Spa Water

Spa water isn't just for relaxation, it's for weight loss, too.
My version will help you look rockin' in your short shorts,
as it's packed with nothing but ingredients *proven* to help you
de-bloat and so, it's guaranteed to float your boat.

SERVES 2 (OR 1 WITH REFILLS)

24 ounces hot water

1 or 2 green tea bags

1 ginger tea bag or a chunk of fresh ginger

½ lemon, cut into chunks

½ lime, cut into chunks

¼ orange, cut into chunks

1 tablespoon apple cider vinegar

Stevia to taste

1. Boil the water, then pour it into a pitcher. Add the green tea
   and ginger tea and let steep for 10 to 15 minutes.

2. Add the lemon, lime, orange, apple cider vinegar, and stevia, give it a shake, and let it chill in your fridge until cold.
   Sip throughout the day.

Food for When You Move Your Body

Whether you lift, stretch, or run, eating plants can help you do it better. They give your body energy versus robbing it of energy like crap foods do. When you eat processed food, your body needs to work hard to figure out how in good god to break it down, digest it, and get it the eff out of there. When you eat plants, your body turns into Anna Wintour's assistant and takes care of business in a flash so you're left with a ton of energy to do your favorite activities, and recover from them, too. Recovery counts as a duty on your body's to-do list. And all this, in a nutshell, is why plants will help you be better at fitness. And lawn mowing.

WHEN YOU WORKED OUT HARD AND CAN BARELY LIFT YOUR ARMS OR EVEN SIT ON THE TOILET

I already spoke (on page 43) about why—while perhaps misguided or underinformed—the folks who are constantly asking "But where do you get your protein?" are not totally wrong. But with these post-workout treats I can show, not just tell, how I consume my post-workout plant protein super well. *(Apparently writing about being strong like Zeus turns me in Dr. Seuss.)*

Heaven in My Apartment Protein Smoothie (Chocolate or Vanilla)

There's a plant food mecca here in NYC that makes a smoothie called "Heaven on Earth," and I love it so much that I have to force myself to not overdo it lest I bore myself of something I adore. When I trial-and-errored my way into re-creating it in my own blender, I made sure to make it customizable so I wouldn't pull another "All About That Bass" fiasco (yes, I may have burned out on that one). Vary your base and your other ingredients, because, thanks to the plant protein for your muscles, dates for your glycogen stores, cinnamon for inflammation, and almond butter for your satiety, whatever combo you choose will be "All About That Workout Recovery."

MAKES 1 SMOOTHIE

1 cup frozen cauliflower florets or riced (or ½ cup frozen cauliflower plus ½ cup coarsely chopped frozen banana)

2 Medjool dates, pitted

1 scoop plant-based chocolate (or vanilla) protein powder

1 tablespoon almond butter, peanut butter, cashew butter, or tahini

¾ teaspoon cinnamon

1 cup almond milk or other plant-based milk

½ teaspoon cacao powder (optional; best if using chocolate protein powder)

1 handful of spinach (optional, but why not?)

Add the cauliflower, dates, protein powder, almond butter, cinnamon, almond milk, cacao powder, and spinach to a high-speed blender and blend until creamy dreamy.

AFTER [PARTY] THOUGHT:

That's not a typo: Try frozen cauliflower instead of bananas if you're cutting down on sugar or just want to mix it up. Cauliflower will put the *smooth* into your smoothie and make you feel nice and have a full belly thanks to its freakish quantities of fiber.

LEFTOVERS ARE THE BESTOVERS:

One recipe tester blended a double batch and froze half in an ice cube tray, and then re-blended it the next day in a flash. Smart girl.

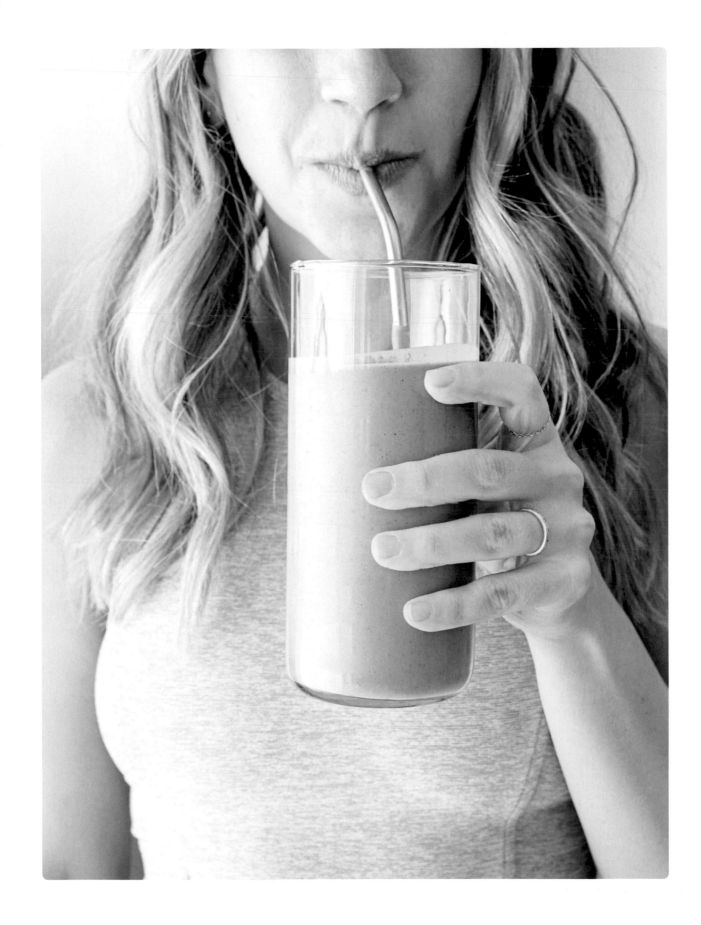

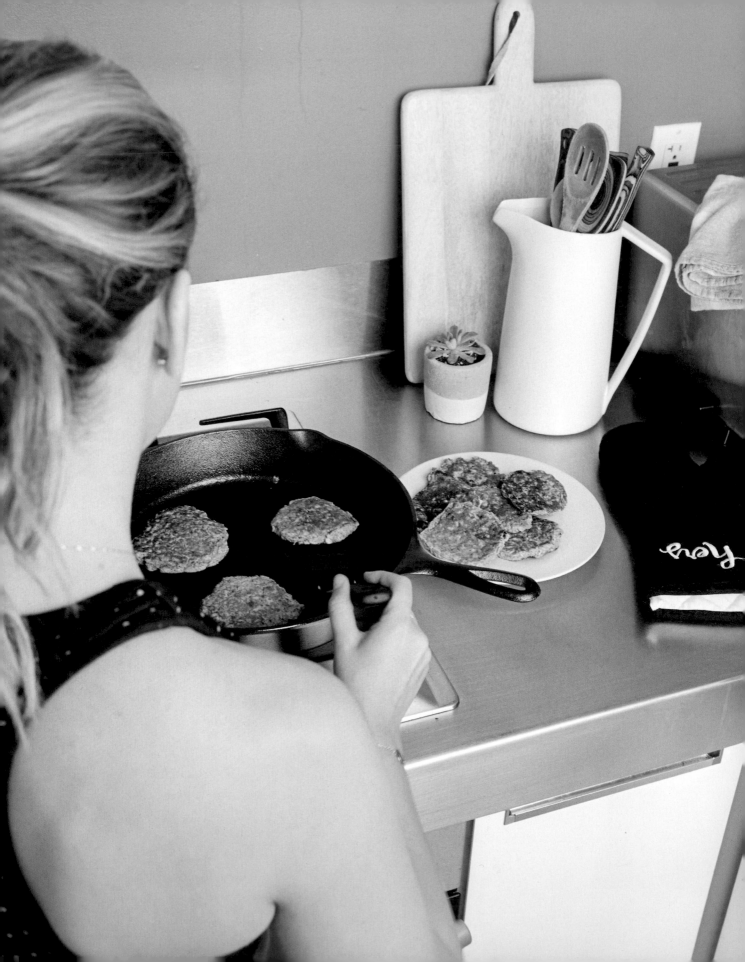

Party in Your Plant-Protein Pancakes

These pancakes are the antidote to pancake belly. It wasn't until I started making them that I learned that pancakes *don't* have to be a precursor to a nap. Instead, they'll leave you feeling energized and satisfied. Not only are they my go-to post-workout breakfast but also my preferred fuel for long flights and car rides, meetings, and even an occasional "emergency" dinner.

Keep your taste buds on their toes by mixing up the flavors. I often add a capful of an extract (almond, lemon, strawberry, or vanilla), and top with different fruits and nut butters.

SERVES 1 OR 2

1 tablespoon flax meal

½ ripe banana, mashed with a fork

1 scoop brown rice protein powder (¼ cup)

6 tablespoons plain, unsweetened almond, oat, or other plant-based milk

¼ teaspoon cinnamon

½ teaspoon baking powder

½ cup rolled oats

Plant-derived sweetener to taste, such as some drops or sprinkles of stevia (liquid or powdered), 1 to 2 teaspoon of maple syrup, or agave

Coconut oil spray coconut oil, to grease the griddle

Nut butter, coconut/almond yogurt, fruit, sweeteners (optional toppings)

1. Combine the flax meal and 2 tablespoons warm water in a small bowl or cup with a fork, then set aside for 5 minutes or until it becomes a gel. Gently stir every minute or so.

2. Mix the banana, protein powder, almond milk, cinnamon, oats, and sweetener together in a large bowl. Stir in the flax egg.

3. Spritz a griddle or pan with coconut oil spray, or melt a dollop or two of coconut oil in your pan and turn the heat to medium-low or medium.

4. Hover your hand over the griddle. When it feels nice 'n toasty, it's ready!

5. Use a ¼-cup measuring cup to add the batter to the griddle. Cook for 4 to 5 minutes, until the facedown side is golden (take a lil peek with your spatula).

6. Flip them, then reduce the heat a smidge. Cook for another 5 minutes, until the other side is golden, too.

continued

7. Remove from the griddle and eat as is, or top them with nut butter, coconut/almond yogurt, fruit, and sweetener.

AFTER [PARTY] THOUGHT:

If you're down to eat eggs, then turn down the flax egg and make this recipe with ⅓ cup of egg whites instead. Omit the almond milk, too.

LEFTOVERS ARE THE BESTOVERS:

These pancakes freeze like a dream. Which your life will feel like when you're too tired or lazy or short on time to make breakfast and then you remember you have frozen pancakes to defrost and devour.

WHEN YOU'RE ABOUT TO WORK OUT HARD AND YOU NEED MORE THAN A PUMP-UP PLAYLIST

Usually all I need is a solid blasting of "Cotton Eye Joe" to get me in the mood, but, for the days that a Jock Jam won't do the trick, I fall back on this sip and snack for that.

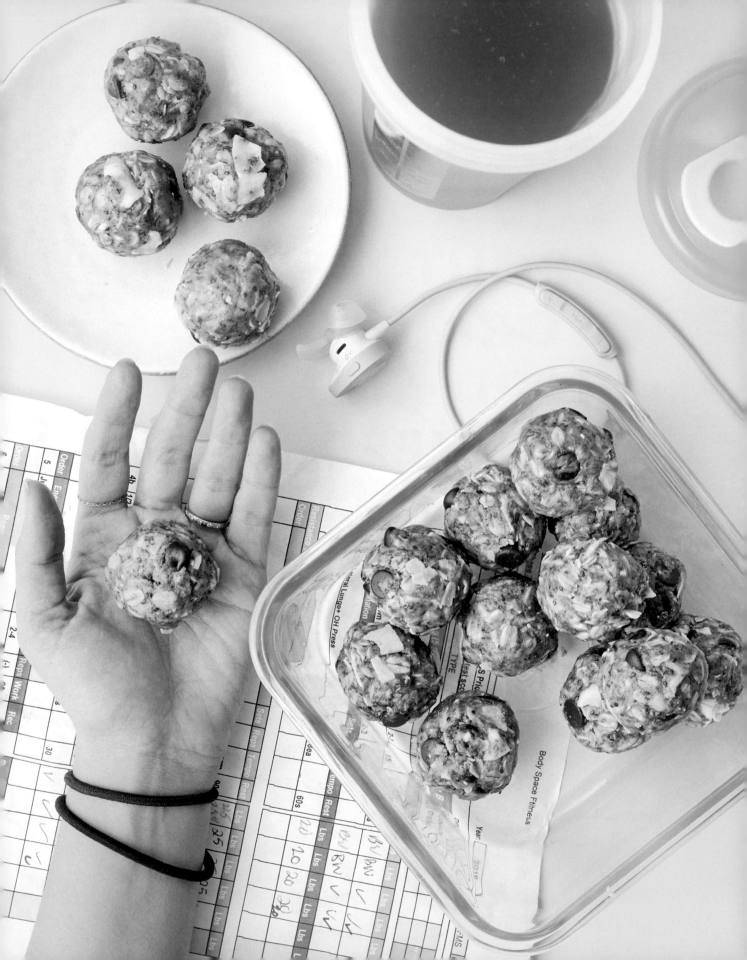

Super[food] Pre-Party in Your Mouth Snack Balls

I begged for this recipe, I'll have you know. They're sold at my favorite spot on Nantucket (an island off the coast of Massachusetts—hi, Lemon Press!), and I've always mourned their absence in my life when summer vacation comes to a close. When Lemon Press catered our joint bachelor/bachelorette party, I got to see firsthand how even our non-health-conscious friends were pounding these superfood snacks one to one with beers. If these could rev our besties up for the festivities, they will rev you up for workouts, too.

MAKES ABOUT 20 BALLS, DEPENDING ON SIZE

1 cup rolled oats

1 tablespoon chia seeds

½ cup flax meal

Pinch of salt

⅔ cup unsweetened coconut flakes or shredded coconut

½ cup chocolate chips

¼ cup plus 1 tablespoon raw honey

½ cup plus 1 tablespoon peanut butter

1 teaspoon vanilla extract

1. Combine the oats, chia seeds, flax meal, salt, coconut flakes, chocolate chips, honey, peanut butter, and vanilla in a large bowl and mix together thoroughly. Get in there with clean hands.

2. Refrigerate the batter for 30 minutes to firm everything up.

3. Use your hands to roll the batter into small balls. In my kitchen, 2 tablespoons = 1 ball.

4. Store these cuties covered in the fridge or covered at room temperature for quick-and-easy mouth-poppin'.

GREATorade

For Miss Massively Competitive over here, the only fun part about getting subbed out in high school basketball was having a break to chug some red Gatorade. In hindsight, it's a good thing I played most of the game (booya!) because that stuff contains not one semblance of real food. I've since shifted from three-point shooting to three-mile running, and have shifted my preferred power drink, too. GREATorade gets its flavor from real fruit juice, its sugar from real honey, its electrolytes from real coconut water (and a pinch of sea salt), plus it gives you an energizing boost from pure green tea. It can replenish kids (nix the caffeine), teens, and adults and would be silly to waste dumping on the head of a winning coach.

MAKES ABOUT 2 QUARTS

1½ cups coconut water

1½ cups pre-brewed iced green or yerba maté tea

1 cup 100% fruit juice, such as watermelon, pineapple, mango, or cranberry

2 tablespoons raw honey

¼ teaspoon sea salt

2 to 3 teaspoons freshly squeezed lemon or lime juice (optional)

In a 2-quart pitcher, stir together the coconut water, tea, and fruit juice.
Stir in the honey and salt until it's dissolved.
Stir in 4 cups water and add the lemon or lime juice to taste, if desired.
Serve chilled.

A Cravings Crash Course

CRAVINGS, YOUR SIXTH SENSE

My cravings get the best of me!" "Plants don't fulfill my cravings!" "It gives me anxiety to think that I will have to suppress my cravings forever!" The way people talk about cravings implies they're an all-powerful force, like the dead people that Haley Joel Osment cannot not see in The Sixth Sense.

The thing is, I believe cravings *are* your sixth sense, but not a legit scapegoat for eating an entire bag of chocolate chips. They're also not a sign of weakness. Just like Haley Joel Osment was able to talk to the ghost of a young Mischa Barton whose mom had poisoned her and then expose said mom, saving Mischa's younger sister from being her next victim, you can talk to your cravings and save *yourself* from being a supersize bag of kettle corn's next target.

Cravings are our body's way of telling us something. They're like our internal Twitter. We have to stop scrolling our feed and actually pause and read or listen to what our cravings are saying.

Here's how these conversations usually go:

> "Hey cutie! (Positive self-talk is always a plus.) What am I craving?"

Something sweet, salty, creamy, chocolatey, carby? Or something specific*?

*I pay extra-close attention to specific cravings. If it's a brand or flavor of a bar or a processed "healthy" snack that I'm dreaming of multiple days in a row, I take that as a sign that I'm overdoing it and even creating an addiction. If it's an apple or a bowl of carrot sticks, I take that as a sign that I've been feeding my body well. If you're *for reals* hungry, you won't foodiscriminate—pretty much anything will satisfy you. But if you've got a *craving,* only a specific food or type of food will calm ya down.

> ### "What am I up to?"
> Am I browsing cookie recipes on Pinterest and shocker! Am now craving cookies? If so, I know this is a BS craving and I laugh at myself, curse Pinterest, and go cuddle with my dog. Or am I trying to finish some important emails and can't stop salivating for something salty? That might mean I'm dehydrated so time to chugalug some agua.

We can have memory cravings, too. My second semester sophomore year of college, I would watch *How I Met Your Mother* while getting ready for class and eating toaster waffles. The next semester I moved to California, got enlightened about plants, and switched my breakfasts to smoothies, but to this day, every time I start to bop to that *HIMYM* theme song, I start aggressively craving those toaster waffles, too.

"What's going on right now?"
Am I stressed? Or lonely? Bored? Sad? Nervous? Mad? You may be craving stuff to fill an emotional void, but spoiler alert: It won't work.

Tired?
Like a car, we can run out of gas and need to pull over from whatever we're doing to refill our energy sources, and that can lead to cravings.

Way past overdue for lunch?
You might be focused on finishing work so you can take a half-day Friday, but your body didn't forget about its need for fuel.

Could I be dehydrated?
Thirst is a tricky sensation—we often don't experience it until we're already on the verge of dehydration, which can be masked under a feeling of mild hunger.

Have I eaten lots of CRAP lately?
Eating crap often leads to our bodies wanting us to eat more crap. If your diet of late has been bereft of nutrients, you may crave short-term energy boosts like caffeine and sugar.

PMS?
If you go through it, you know that these cyclical cravings can be Pretty Massively Strong.

Did I work out like a beast a few hours ago?
Demanding a lot from your body (in the form of long runs, sweaty yoga, or heavy weights) means you need extra nutritional love.

Am I feeling flipping fabulous and want to celebrate?
Call it self-sabotage or call it one of the weirdest habits of human nature, but sometimes when things are going swell, we'll latch on to a boohockey belief that we don't deserve to be happy and sabotage ourselves by popping Pop-Tarts and sucking down Oreo sleeves.

In these moments, I imagine myself eating a couple of different things. Like looking in my closet to consider how three different sweaters would look with this one pair of jeans, I'll look in my mind and imagine how an apple, for example, would taste, or a homemade matcha latte, or even a leftover bowl of chili. Usually, the answer is crystal clear.

ONE EXCEPTION: MY TWO-BLOCK RULE

I'm blessed to live in a neighborhood with multiple artisanal vegan ice cream options within a five-block radius of my home. Considering I still have scars from when I used to hack open a coconut, scrape out the meat, and use an ice cream maker to make my own, this is as shocking as it must have been when TVs went from black and white to color. And since ice cream is my favorite thing in the world, I find myself craving it a lot. I know better than to keep pints in my freezer—even my homemade kale ice cream barely lasts twenty-four hours—so I make myself adhere to a two-block rule. Ready?

I don't GO OUT OF MY WAY to satisfy a craving. Way too many times when I first moved to NYC, I found myself thinking that a vegan cupcake sounded nice, and before I knew what was going on, I was bra-lessly meandering over to the city's then best vegan bakery eight blocks away. After I moved apartments, I realized how inappropriately committed I had been to fueling that particular sugar addiction and the rule was born: If I have to go out of my way to get my fix, then it's a no-go. No food should have that kind of power over me. A clean craving never causes us to zombie walk anywhere in indoor clothes. Or manic panic pull off the side of the road to satisfy it.

Your "two blocks" may be a long detour to that bakery. It may be a $20 delivery charge because a $5 cup of ice cream doesn't meet the delivery minimum. It may be running out to the grocery store for chips because your body *needs them now*. Whatever your particular boondoggle, notice the difference between a calm craving and a crazy craving, because that's really what we're talking about here. Crazy cravings brainwash you to drop your kid in day care so you can get your fajitas fix, while calm cravings inspire you to ask yourself the aforementioned questions.

How to give in to all your cravings in 1–2–3–4:

Pause before mouth stuffing begins and simply notice you're having a craving.

Brainstorm the healthiest and low-hanging-fruitiest way to satisfy it.

Eat that.

If there's no obvious healthy substitution and you don't need to go out of the equivalent two-block radius to satisfy it, then do it with a damn smile because stress is worse for you than a pesticide.

HOW TO CRAVE MORE PLANTS

There's certainly not a shortage of healthy recipes around, yet so many of my clients, family, and friends still struggle to eat well. I eventually realized that it's not always about lack of food knowledge, it's sometimes about the mind-set. Here are some tried-and-true ways to shift your mindset to help you *want* to eat more plants.

REMEMBER THAT FOOD IS FUEL.

Food gives us energy: energy to function, to work, to run errands, and to do all of the things in life we love to do, whether that's traveling, stand-up paddleboard, or playing Ping-Pong. Since they are jam-packed with natural nutrients and are easily digestible, the energy in plants shoots right into our bodies. When we start to think of food as fuel, things like a midnight snack becomes unnecessary (who needs fuel to sleep?) and a healthy breakfast is an obvious choice (who doesn't need fuel to have a tremendous day?).

YOU CAN'T BE HEALTHY WITHOUT BEING HAPPY. BUT YOU ALSO CAN'T BE HAPPY WITHOUT BEING HEALTHY.

Happiness and health go hand in hand. Like sushi and chopsticks, summer and Banana Ice Cream (page 110) or smoothies and mason jars, you can't have one without the other. If you're choking down a salad with anger, resentment, and jealousy of your dining companion's double bacon cheeseburger, you're doing more harm than good. Negative emotions, especially while eating, can cause digestive distress, reducing your ability to fully absorb nutrients. So instead of forcing yourself to eat more plants, remind yourself that you're eating more plants so that you can live a healthier and thus a happier overall life. Sure, the guy next to you is inhaling his juicy burger, but will he feel energized and satisfied later? I think not. But you, my plant-eating friend, will feel phenomenal. Eat that salad with all the joy and appreciation you can muster. Your future self will thank you.

ASK YOURSELF: "IS 30 SECONDS OF FLAVOR WORTH HOW I'LL FEEL IN AN HOUR?"

This is a personal favorite of mine. Asking this question before reaching for that bread basket or ordering dessert or getting that third glass of wine has proven time and time again to help me make the wisest decision for my body. That dinner roll would give me maybe thirty seconds of palate pleasure, but would leave me feeling yucky, bloated, and unsatisfied just minutes later. Tap into your body's inner wisdom and use that to guide your decisions. When you gleefully pick the fruity sorbet over the decadent cake because you know how sluggish the latter would make you feel in an hour, you'll experience pride unlike anything else.

THE MORE ALIVE YOUR FOOD IS, THE MORE ALIVE IT'LL MAKE YOU FEEL.

Raw, a.k.a. living, plants (fruits, veggies, nuts, and seeds) have all their nutrients intact. Because they haven't been heated, they come with naturally occurring digestive enzymes, which help our bodies break them down and absorb their nutrients with little to no effort. The less energy we spend on digesting, the more energy we have for exercise, spending time with loved ones, or figuring out that damn Sudoku.

ONE TASTE ISN'T GOING TO KILL YOU. (THIS WORKS BOTH WAYS.)

You're at a wedding. The non-gluten-free, non-dairy-free, non-refined-sugar-free three-tiered wedding cake is staring you in the face and you can't even concentrate on doing the cha-cha slide without knowing what it tastes like. *Have a bite.* And really take a moment to enjoy it!

Same thing when trying a new plant-based dish. Steamed kale isn't the most attractive on the plate. But in this case, taking one bite can shatter any fears and misconceptions—and maybe you've found a new fave meal.

NOTHING TASTES AS GOOD AS BEING HEALTHY FEELS.

Cliché? Maybe. But true? Definitely. Doesn't matter how good that deep-dish pizza might taste in the moment, it can't possible taste as good as living long enough to see your grandkids grow up, having energy to travel around the world, or maintaining the mental clarity to excel in your career feels.

GIVE YOURSELF EMOTIONAL REASONS TO EAT WELL.

Visualize yourself skiing down the mountains of Colorado, feeling light and comfortable riding the waves on the Cape, walking your daughter down the aisle—always feeling strong and vibrant. When you give yourself emotional whys, and pull those reasons up in moments of temptation, often the big picture will inspire you to push aside the cheese puffs.

HELLO, BODY, IT'S ME, TALIA

"Listen to your body" is the most frustrating advice on the advice circuit right now. (Second place is: to consult an astrologist over a therapist.) Listening to your body is far from a science. It's more like interpreting a poem. Or Drake lyrics. Or a Jackson Pollock painting. (Whom I'm not related to in case you've been wondering.)

All I can tell you is this: Food makes you feel stuff. That is a fact. The way we physically feel is not arbitrary. Food makes us feel good stuff, bad stuff, energetic stuff, sluggish stuff. If you can accept that the same way we all know that music makes us feel stuff, you can begin to truly listen. And just like music, the volume of your feelings can vary. The more you tune in after a meal to figure out how you're doing, the louder your "listen to your body" volume will become. But like you intentionally put your headphones on your head to listen to music, you've got to intentionally listen to your body, too.

Once you notice, you won't be able to *un-notice.* You'll become empowered. You'll know that how you feel is up to you. Before eating, I always ask myself, "Does this meal match how I want to feel?" Wanna feel energized? Eat some fruit. Wanna feel sluggish and stuck on the couch? Eat some fries. It's that simple.

And there are times that I am on board with feeling kind of gross! In the winter, I'm often perfectly happy eating something heavy that sinks me right down. The important thing is that it's a *conscious* decision, and that more often I choose something that's going to make me light up. And you already know what food that is: plants.

WTF IS WILLPOWER? AND HOW YOU CAN GET IT

Remember a million years ago I asked you to get clear on the consequences of not eating right? I used the analogy about how thinking about the negative consequences of not having a charged phone (like tragically not being able to Instagram what you ate for dinner) makes you want to always have a charged phone, I said that getting clear on your consequences of not eating plants will help you always plan to eat more plants. That's willpower, baby. Willpower is the *power* of saying, "I'll honor my why." The more you bring that into your consciousness, the more you will have.

Think about how many times you've lied, snuck around, and done weird stuff to get something you wanted. Maybe you have a system to sneakily text your boyfriend at work, or you've quietly taken a call for a job you really want from the bathroom of your job that you really hate. When you have your mind and heart set on something, you made it happen.

It is the same with food. If you truly want to feel well, you'll eat well. That's all there is to it.

THE EMPOWERED NO

Okay, there's a little more to it. There's the empowered no, something I am very obsessed with. Saying no gets a bad rap. It makes us feel like we're boring, restricted, or missing out. But if your friend asked you to go skydiving and since you're deathly afraid of heights, you wouldn't hesitate to respond with a big fat *nah*. Or if your office crush asked if you'd like a drag of his cigarette but you don't smoke, it'd be no struggle to turn it down.

The empowered no for food operates under the same principle. When you're presented with a bowl of Funyons, if you know (since you listen to your body and are aware that food makes you feel stuff) that grabbing a handful will make the moments after eating them less than fun, it's no problem at all to demur. I whip out empowered no's all the time, like when presented with Jell-O shots, oysters, or caviar.

My mother once said something about willpower I'll never forget. We were eating lunch with my sister before going to try on my wedding dress. My mom had just tried on her own dress for my wedding and wasn't completely over the moon with how it hugged her sixty-five-year-old hips. Over her bowl of risotto, she said, "I think I've aged out of willpower." I reminded her of the same thing I just told you: Willpower simply means saying, "I'll honor my why." Perhaps she had lost touch with her why over the years, when she cared more for her daughters than herself. Or maybe her desire to feel comfortable in her jeans faded with twenty years of marriage. But later that night at dinner, seemingly out of the blue, her willpower reappeared in full force when she boldly passed on the bread basket.

WHY BEING A PICKY EATER IS BS

My favorite soapbox to get on when I speak in public is about how not liking healthy food is BS. This is the biggest hit with college students, but it works for anyone over the age of twenty-one.

Take a moment to consider the first time you sipped alcohol. I want you to be real with yourself: Did you like it?

I'm not talking about if you liked how it helped you dance confidently at Suzie's bat mitzvah, or encouraged you to kiss that hottie at the Super Bowl, or made you pee your pants laughing during Pictionary. I'm asking if you liked how it tasted.

I'm positive that your answer is no: You did not like that first sip, or even the twelfth one. But you tried it again, right? (Even if you don't drink alcohol for whatever reason, stick with me for one more sec.) Because you loved how it made you *feel*. You loved being silly and confident and goofy. So over time your taste buds adapted because you wanted to keep the fun rolling.

I'll argue till the cabbage ferments that you can do this same thing with healthy food: If you can adapt your buds to booze, you can do the same for healthy foods. When you start to notice how certain foods make you feel, you will want to keep going. Your taste buds will learn to play along. When you were an alcohol newbie, you went for that Mike's Hard Lemonade type stuff, right? Or Manischewitz? Some of the sweetest stuff on earth. After a while of drinking that alcoholic sugar, you started being okay with a vodka soda, or a sav blanc. Same thing can happen for you and green juice. Why not start getting a healthy green juice with loads of pineapple in it? It'll be super sweet, but you'll still reap its positive effects. After a few weeks, you'll be able to try green juice with a pear or apple, and then no fruit whatsoever.

Or, fine, you've never liked broccoli. Cover it with a creamy sauce. Go on, eat it a few times a week under a puddle of ranch or cheese. Then one day, try the broccoli without it—instead, roast and smother it in Red Peppa Pesto (page 209). I guarantee your taste buds will be on board.

And just remember: The grosser it looks, the less gross it's gonna make you feel. That's how I got through those first few green smoothies. As I started to feel better and more energized from my daily green treats, I started to look forward to my gross daily dose of liquid health.

WHEN YOU'RE PMSING. OR IT'S VALENTINE'S DAY. OR YOU'RE JUST CRAVING CHOCOLATE.

Chocolate cravings happen. Quite frequently for some of us. Whether there's a rhyme or no reason, you can satisfy even the most hardcore chocolate hankering with these two recipes.

Wussup, Chocolate-Covered Chia Jam Cups

I learned how to DIY chocolate peanut butter cups when the only option on the market had a name that rhymed with Zeese's. Considering that growing up I'd trade every single Halloween candy in my pillowcase for this particular treat, it was a nonstarter to consider cutting peanut butter cups from my life. Now that there are plenty of less unhealthy versions on the market, I've updated my version by stuffing them with real-fruity chia jam. If you're a fan of chocolate-covered fruit, you'll be a super fan of these elegant cups.

MAKES 12 TO 15 SMALL CUPS

CHIA JAM

1 cup frozen fruit (cherries, raspberries, blueberries, strawberries)

1 tablespoon chia seeds, plus more to sprinkle on top if desired

1½ tablespoons honey or maple syrup

½ teaspoon freshly squeezed lemon juice

DISH

2 cups chocolate chips (dark or semisweet)

1 teaspoon coconut oil

Pinch of sea salt, plus more to sprinkle on top if desired

12 to 15 little paper cups

1. Make the chia jam: In a small pot on the stove over medium heat, add the frozen fruit. Once the fruit begins to melt and get a little juicy, add the chia seeds, honey, and lemon juice. Reduce the heat to low and cook for 1 minute, stirring frequently.

2. Turn off the heat and stir some more—you want the chia seeds to expand and become jam-like. Remove from the stove.

3. Melt the chocolate in a microwave or in a double boiler (see page 79). Stir in the coconut oil until it melts and add a pinch of salt until everything blends together. Set aside.

4. Line a mini muffin baking tin with baking cups. Place ½ teaspoon of chocolate in each cup, then 1 teaspoon of the chia jam, then ½ teaspoon of melted chocolate to fill the cup. Repeat until you've run out of ingredients. Sprinkle a pinch of salt or chia seeds on top of each cup if you like.

5. Leave the cups out for about 1 hour for the chocolate to harden. (In chocolate emergencies, you can put them into your freezer for about 8 minutes.)

6. Peel and eat and store leftovers in the fridge. Store the jam in a jar in the fridge, too. It keeps for about 1 week.

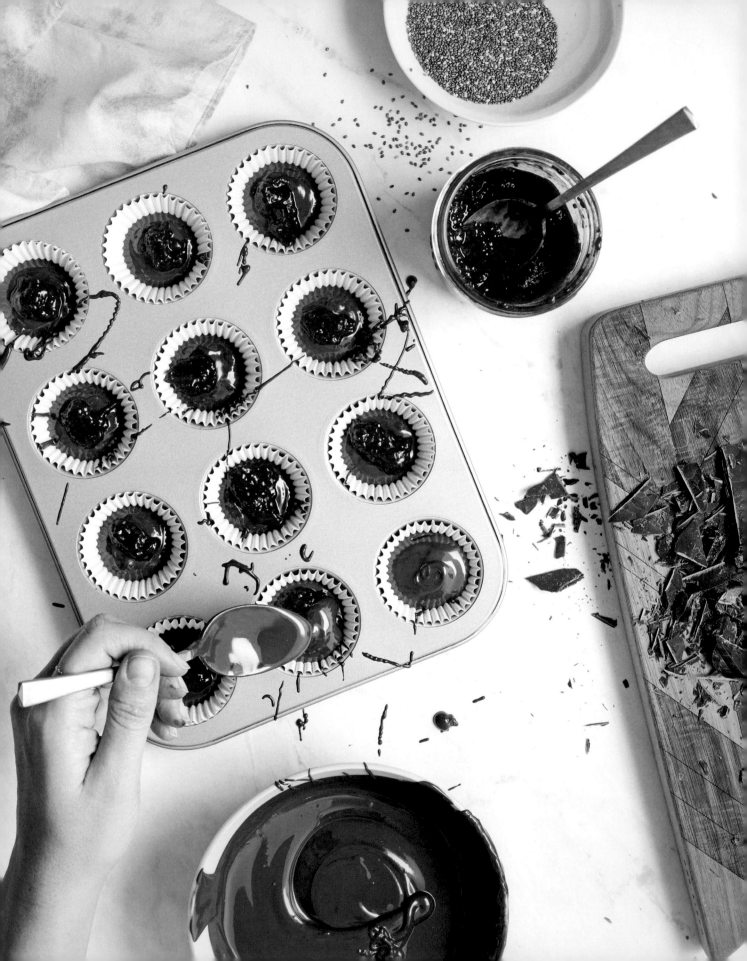

LEFTOVERS ARE THE BESTOVERS:

It'd be unfair for you to limit this jam to these cups. That'd be as tragic as if Justin had limited himself to 'NSync. Since this jam is bound to be your jam, make it a fridge staple to use on toasts (Toast Twenty Ways, page 206), pancakes (Party in Your Plant-Protein Pancakes, page 299), or Gift-Worthy Granola (page 263).

AFTER [PARTY] THOUGHT:

Want to make the OG cups? Forget about the chia jam and fill the cups with 1 teaspoon of nut butter instead.

Cacao Potahto

Maybe you thought that cacao and cocoa were like grey & gray, donut & doughnut, disc & disk: same difference. I'm sorry, but you thought wrong. CacAO is the raw version of chocolate. Cacao grows on trees in football-like colorful pods. Inside are huge seeds called cacao beans even though they're seeds (just go with it). If you dry the beans, remove their skin, and press them, they crumble into nibs. Grind up the nibs and you get cacao powder.

It's loaded with antioxidants, keeping you and your skin young, your cholesterol low, your heart healthy, and your blood clean. It's also a high-magnesium food, which helps you sleep, have bowel movements, and keep your muscles relaxed. It's rich in calcium and iron, keeping your blood and your bones strong. Cacao is energy boosting (because it's got caffeine) and happiness-increasing (because it releases serotonin). And love, it's an aphrodisiac.

So consuming cacao is how you can justify calling chocolate "healthy." And these crumbs (my high-in-plant-protein, quinoa-based cacao granola, which'll turn your almond milk as chocolatey as your Cocoa Krispies did back in the day) are how you can justify eating chocolate for breakfast.

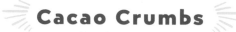

Cacao Crumbs

MAKES ABOUT 4 CUPS

1½ cups rolled oats

1 cup quinoa (dry, raw, not rinsed)

2 tablespoons chia seeds

¼ cup cacao powder

½ teaspoon sea salt

¼ cup shredded unsweetened coconut

2 tablespoons coconut oil

2 tablespoons almond or cashew butter (or peanut butter, but then your granola will have a peanut butter flavor versus the other two nut butters, which are more neutral tasting)

¼ cup maple syrup

1 teaspoon vanilla extract

Almond milk or almond or coconut milk yogurt, for serving (optional)

1. Preheat the oven to 350°F.
2. In a large bowl, mix together the oats, quinoa, chia seeds, cacao powder, salt, and coconut.
3. In a small saucepan over medium heat, combine the coconut oil, almond butter, maple syrup, and vanilla and stir to melt until no lumps remain.
4. Pour the wet ingredients over the dry ingredients. Mix well.
5. Spread the mixture on a rimmed baking sheet and put into the oven for 12 minutes.
6. After 12 minutes, remove from the oven, move it around with a spatula, and return it to the oven for another 2 minutes.
7. Remove and let cool. Enjoy with almond milk, mixed into almond or coconut milk yogurt, or just by the spoonful.

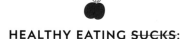

HEALTHY EATING ~~SUCKS~~:

"The only bad thing is that I don't have a shovel to shovel it into my mouth faster." **—JN**

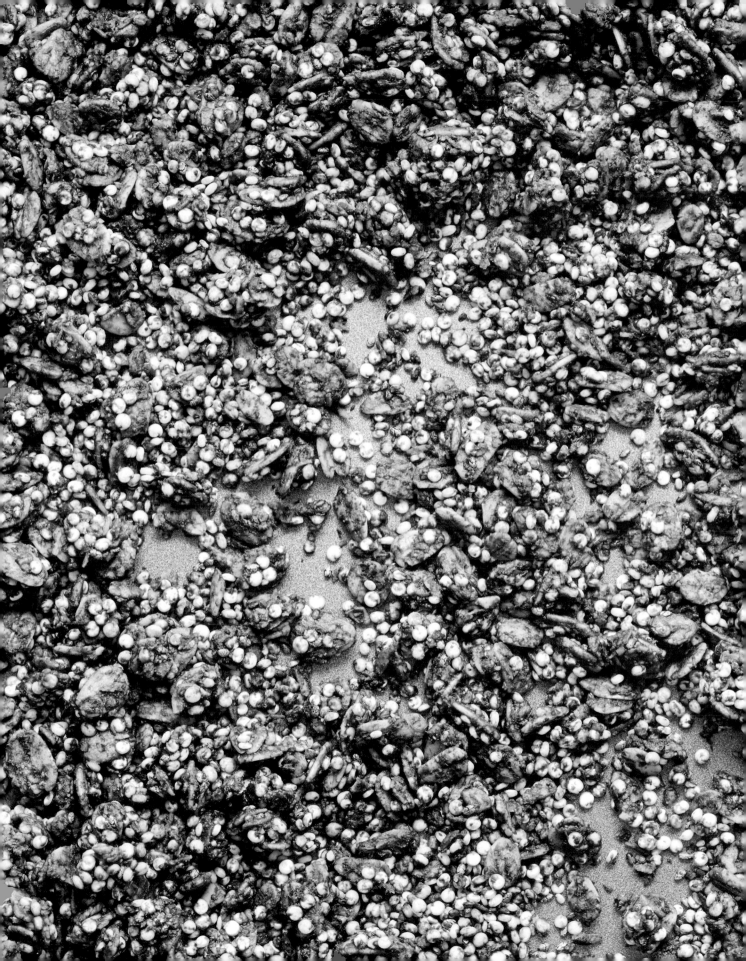

Digestion

When a new "cast" starts on *The Bachelor*, all the women get brief online bios with unflattering head shots. One of the questions each has to answer is "What's your biggest date fear?"

I was perusing the site a few years back, expecting to read the things like "losing a fake eyelash" or "tripping" or "the guy calling me the name of the other redhead on the show." But what I saw in overwhelming volume was "having stomach issues and clogging up the toilet," "gas and violent diarrhea," "getting stomach cramps," and "diarrhea" (yes—it was there twice). I thought, "Wow! So many people struggle with digestive distress," "Tummy problems are a big deal," and "That bachelor is screwed if his potential wives don't read this chapter."

If you're anything like those contestants, or even if you're the exact opposite, I imagine that you struggle with digestive issues on occasion as well. This might mean you get gassy or bloated, have indigestion or pain, constipation or diarrhea. If you're experiencing any of these on a regular basis (two times or more per week), your tummy ain't happy—and I can imagine that you ain't so happy, either.

I feel your pain. Literally.

I struggled with life-impeding digestive issues for eight years. EIGHT.

That's like watching the first *Hunger Games* movie thirty thousand times back to back. That's a lotta Jennifer Lawrence. And a lotta tummyaches.

As you know by now, I healed myself. And you can, too.

THE IBS BS

As I mentioned before, in my world, an "IBS" diagnosis is total BS. It's a catch-all term that doctors like to throw around when they don't know what the heck is wrong. It's like seeing a "damaged" tag on a jacket in a store and not knowing if it has a stain, a rip, a snag, a burn, a missing button, or one sleeve shorter than the other—just that there's something off.

The good news about being told you have IBS is that it means you probably don't have anything more serious. High five! That's worth celebrating. The bad news is that it means you'll have to figure out how to make your uniquely damaged jacket wearable. Here's what worked for me:

TREATING MY TUMMY LIKE A TODDLER
Like ignoring a screaming child in a grocery store, it's impossible to ignore a sensitive stomach in a work meeting. But just like cursing a screaming child, telling them,

"I wish you were never born!" or "Why are you *my* child?!" wouldn't make you parent of the year, cursing your sensitive stomach won't make you any healthier. The biggest mental and emotional shift I experienced was when I started treating my body like a toddler, with patience and compassion and unconditional love. You can't choose if your kid is scared of clowns, same way as I couldn't choose if my way of processing the world was almost entirely through my gut, and the moment I had that epiphany, everything changed.

I passed this (arguably weird) philosophy to my client Tracy, who immediately took to it and named her stomach "Timothy." But weirdness works, because instead of writing me emails about how her stomach ruined her day or her date or her vacation, she started writing about how poor Timothy had been upset, so she gave him some TLC and he was feeling better. Maybe acceptance is the new Advil.

USING DIGESTIVE ENZYMES LIKE SPANX

Spanx may help you look sleeker in a photo, but it can't change your body—your bone structure, height, or weight and digestive enzymes can't change your digestive system. They won't cure your peanut allergy or make it so that cupcakes don't go straight to your love handles. But, much like Spanx, they can give you an advantage. Digestive enzymes lessen the blow that a few french fries takes on your heartburn, and help you digest that holiday pie a little bit quicker than you would otherwise.

I take and recommend digestive enzymes if you're about to eat something you notoriously don't digest very easily. Again, this doesn't mean if you're lactose intolerant you can just pop a few and enjoy a milk shake, but it does mean that if you're like me and non-gluten-free bread makes you feel nonperfect, but you know you're going to a restaurant that has only sandwiches, taking digestive enzymes before eating might help lessen how lousy you feel.

Digestive enzymes are also like insurance: there to protect you from things you can't anticipate. For example, if I get an unpleasant email just as I'm sitting down to eat dinner. Eating while experiencing negative emotions can affect digestion for the worse, and since I don't want to walk away from dinner angry about the email *and* at my stomach, I'll pop a few digestive enzymes before eating to give me a boost.

They also come in handy when I'm traveling. Traveling takes a tremendous toll on our digestion. The stress, the chaos, the foreign food, time differences, airplane madness, sleep deprivation, dehydration—any of the above can eff up our ability to break down the food we eat.

Take them as close to a meal as possible, but don't stress about it. Let's go back to Spanx. You wouldn't smush yourself into Spanx three hours before a big event, or three hours after. You want the Spanx when you need it the most, during your moment in the spotlight. Same with digestive enzymes—aim for the moment you dive in to those fries. If you forget, midway through or even a few minutes after will still help.

FOCUSING ON WHAT I THINK WHILE I FORK

I've said this a half-dozen ways already, but I'll write it again: Our thoughts can tick off our tummies. An upset mind = an upset gut. What's happening up north as we glug a smoothie affects how well we receive and process that smoothie.

I used to be baffled about why some days I could eat a green apple with no problem and other days it would make me feel like someone's fingernails were scraping the inside of my gut. And making me bloat. And giving me gas. And overall being a real biotch. I dissected every possibility: Maybe the bad ones had more bruises. Could nonorganic make my stomach hurt? Had I eaten the sticker?

I eventually realized that it wasn't the apple that had changed. What had changed was where my *head* was at—how high my stress levels were; if I was chewing while reflecting on the beauty of today or cursing the terror that was tomorrow. This led me to prioritize my state of mind more than my seasonings. If I'm fighting with Jesse about something dumb that I'm likely absolutely right about, I will delay eating until we're in a good place. If I have a nerve-racking meeting, I won't eat anything substantial until after. Not only that, I learned that my body feels pretty much the same whether I'm freaking out about something incredible or freaking out about something scary, so even moments of awesomeness can cause negative feelings. My environment, energy, and emotions lay the groundwork.

FINDING MY BFFS (BEST FOOD FRIENDS)

You have your best friends, your coziest bad-day sweatshirts, your most beloved "I can walk *and* wear heels" heels. Similarly, I suggest you identify your belly's best food friends. These "safe foods" are those plants that you, through paying attention, have concluded are the easiest for you to eat and feel not terrible in times of turmoil (or titillation). Marry these foods. Buy stock in these foods. Have these foods in your home at all times. Make these foods (for me, they're sweet potatoes, kale, arugula, apples, kombucha, brown rice pasta, and any and all things made from real ginger) the Pam to your Jim.

WHEN YOUR STOMACH HURTS, BUT YOU STILL NEED TO EAT DINNER

This recipe is my stomach's security blanket. Packed with all of my BFFs, I rely on this soul-soothing supper more than I rely on candlelit bubble baths sound-tracked by Ray Lamontagne.

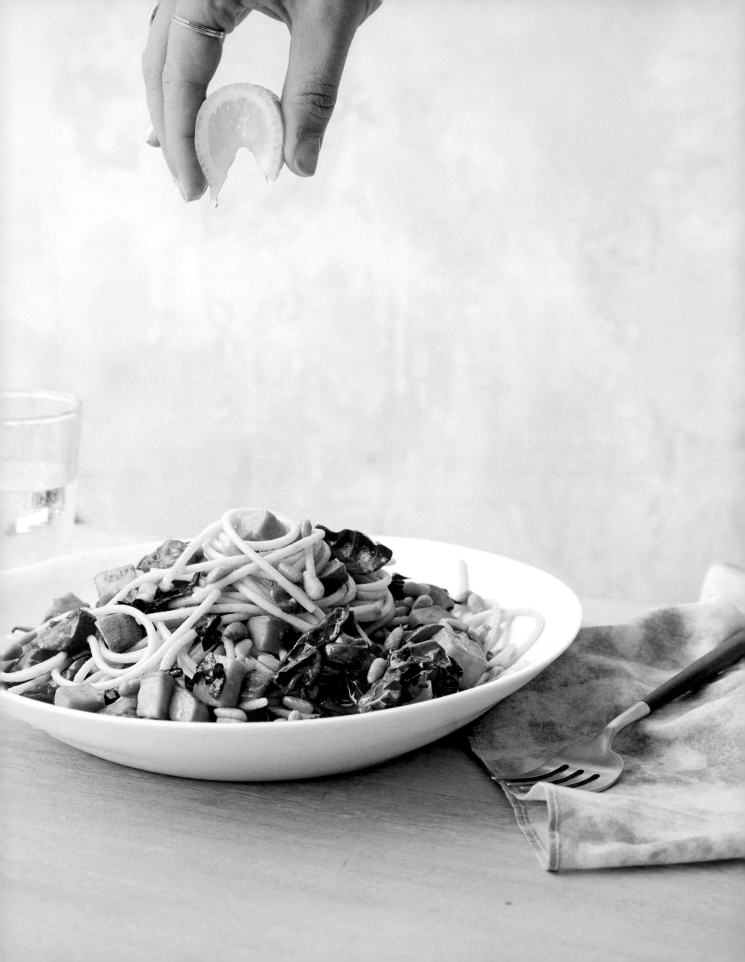

Self-Love Spaghetti

12 to 16 ounces brown rice spaghetti

2 tablespoons extra-virgin olive oil

Sea salt or pink salt to taste

1 large sweet potato, chopped into cubes

¼ cup pine nuts (pumpkin seeds work too) (optional)

1 to 3 garlic cloves, minced

1 small bunch of kale, stems removed and chopped

Red pepper flakes to taste (optional)

Juice of ½ lemon

1. Bring a pot of water to a boil.
2. Add pasta to the pot of boiling water and cook it according to the package's instructions.
3. While it cooks, in a large sauté pan over medium heat, add 1 tablespoon of the olive oil, a few pinches of sea salt, and the sweet potatoes. Cook, uncovered, for 5 minutes. Toss the sweet potatoes around with a wooden spoon, cover the sauté pan with a lid, and cook for 5 more minutes.
4. Place the pine nuts, if using, in a sauté pan over medium heat and toast them for 3 minutes, stirring frequently or shaking the pan until they're golden.
5. Your pasta should be done around now, so drain it and return it to the pot.
6. Add the garlic and kale to the sauté pan with the sweet potatoes, plus the red pepper flakes, if using. Cook for 2 to 3 minutes, until the kale has wilted and turns bright green.
7. Remove from the stove and squeeze lemon juice over the kale.
8. Drizzle the remaining 1 tablespoon olive oil over the cooked pasta, add the sautéed vegetables and pine nuts, and toss. Season with salt to taste and sit down, take deep breaths, think happy thoughts, and serve warm, preferably with ginger tea or ginger kombucha on the side.

General Well-Being and Stuffy Noses

BOOKEND YOUR DAY

We wake up each morning with the best intentions. Well, I'm pretty sure we all do. I can't imagine that anyone wakes up and shouts, "Gooooood morning! It's another beautiful day to make some very unwise, unhealthy decisions! Can't wait to eat lousy to feel lousy! YAAS!"

I think we all want to eat more f*&ing healthy stuff throughout the day. But crap happens. Sometimes your co-workers bring doughnuts to the office, or you meet friends for happy hour, or your roommate orders pizza again. And that's okay. The key to allowing it to happen once in a while without overwhelming you is to bookend your days with plants. That means that you can stress a little less if the middle veers off course.

Kick your day off with one of these two detoxifying, metabolism-revving, fat-burning, skin-beautifying beverages:

1. Lemon water (I'm talking water, preferably warm, plus juice from a lemon)

2. My ACV (apple cider vinegar) drink

3. About 10 ounces water (or coconut water to add sweetness)

4. 2 tablespoons apple cider vinegar

5. About ½ teaspoon cinnamon or 1 scoop of your favorite Greens Powder

6. Stevia or honey to taste

Shake it (like a Polaroid picture) in a shaker cup or blender.

After you flood your cells with one of those two life-giving liquids, it's nice to pump up with plants. Try:

- A green smoothie with plant protein (Heaven in My Apartment Protein Smoothie, page 296)
- Protein pancakes with a few handfuls of fruit on top. (Plus a drizzle of almond or coconut milk yogurt if it makes you happy.) (Party in Your Plant-Protein Pancakes, page 299)

- Fruit-topped overnight oats (Overnight [or Shower Speed] Oats, page 114) or regular cooked plant-packed oatmeal (like Jesse's Secret Creamy, Dreamy Pumpkin Oatmeal on page 84).
- A veggie-packed tofu scramble (Tofu Scramble de Talia, page 185) with a bit of sauerkraut if you wanna give your tummy some bonus TLC. Fab on the side is a slice of gluten-free or whole-grain bread or tortilla with avocado smashed on top and a drizzle of hot sauce.

And remember our Black Turtleneck Theory: It's okay to eat the same thing every day. It's easy enough to mix up the fruits in your green smoothie, play with your oatmeal toppings, and vary the veggies in your tofu scrambles.

Most of us like to end the night with a treat. Routinely that treat is sweet. So if you're ready to wrap up your evening, whatever you had for dinner (which hopefully was plant-packed but sometimes crap does happen), here are some bookends that'll help you sleep tight:

- Banana Ice Cream (page 110)
- Two Snickers Bar Bites (Better Than a Snickers Bar Bites, page 141)
- A commando square (or 2) of the darkest chocolate (highest in cacao) your taste buds will tolerate alongside a glass of almond milk
- Healthy hot cocoa (Hug in a Mug PB Hot Cocoa, page 127)
- Frozen mango chunks right outta the freezer
- Plant-party popcorn (Decked-Out Cinnamon Kettle Corn, page 226) if you're a salty snacker.
- Tea (see "There's a T for Every Y," page 265).

End your days with gut-care, too, which for me means getting magnesium into my body temple. Magnesium, in the form of a fizzy drink, tincture, or supplement, can help you relax, which can in turn help you fall asleep more quickly and then sleep more deeply. It also has an added bonus—better pooping. Magnesium relaxes your colon, which can alleviate constipation if you're prone to that.

If you get into the habit of making a healthy sandwich of your day, your body will get into the habit of feeling great more times than not, and you will naturally start craving more plants so you'll end up having fewer "crap happens" kind of days.

WHEN YOU'RE SICK

If you follow my rule of green thumb of eating more plants than you do crap, your body will more often stay healthy than fall sick. But just like sometimes, even though you triple-checked, your important 6:15 a.m. alarm was set for p.m. and everything goes haywire, sometimes even though you're triple eating your plants, sometimes your immune system can go haywire through no fault of your own. When you're feeling run-down, sniffly-nosed, or scratchy-throated, feed yourself double doses of these recipes to get you back on the road to recovery.

OR: HERE ARE OOMPA LOOMPA FOODS

Why do both of these recipes look like they got aggressive in the spray-tanning booth? But because the most cold-fighting foods look like oompa loompas: Sweet potatoes, oranges, turmeric, ginger, garlic, honey, cinnamon, and cauliflower are all powerful immune boosters.

Magic Mushrooms

Jesse feels about mushrooms the way I feel about aisle seats on fifteen-hour flights. (Disgusted.) Since 'shrooms are practically banned in our home, I turn to mushroom powders. The first time I tried a packet in a glass of hot water, I was skeptical because I run from trendy products like my dog runs from plastic bags, but afterward I felt truly awesome. If there's one craze you want to jump on, let it be this one.

Mushrooms' magical effects aren't a hallucination. Forty percent of pharmaceuticals utilize fungi, including ten out of the top twenty bestselling drugs in the world. Much like the Spice Girls, each has its own unique gift to offer to the world. As a general group, they're known as adaptogens, which are international superstars for your overall immunity. (In short, adaptogens help your body combat stress and fight fatigue.)

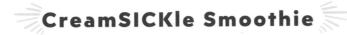

CreamSICKle Smoothie

This is one sick smoothie. Not only, like, *sick, dude,* but for when you're sniffling, sneezing, snotting, coughing, sore throating, hanging over, nauseating, bloating, blah-ing . . . the whole nine. It contains a multitude of immune boosters: orange (loaded with healing vitamin C), ginger (germ killer extraordinaire), turmeric and honey (the queen bees of "heal me" thanks to high levels of nutrients, antioxidants, anti-inflammatory compounds, and phytonutrients), cauliflower (which is not only rich in antibiotics but high in glutathione, which helps fight infections), banana (for hydration and nourishment), and plant protein (to strengthen yourself).

MAKES 1 IMMUNE-BOOSTING SMOOTHIE

1 orange, peeled and coarsely chopped (about 1 cup)

1 tablespoon fresh ginger, peeled and coarsely chopped

1 cup frozen cauliflower florets

½ cup chopped frozen banana slices

½ teaspoon ground turmeric

2 to 4 tablespoons plant-based vanilla protein powder (optional but ideal for feeling full)

½ teaspoon vanilla extract (use 1 full teaspoon if you're not using vanilla protein powder)

½ to 1 teaspoon raw honey

½ cup plant milk (plus 1 to 2 more tablespoons if you, unlike me, prefer thinner smoothies)

1. Add the orange, ginger, cauliflower, banana, turmeric, protein powder, vanilla, honey, and milk to a high-speed blender and blend until creamy.

2. Sip yourself back to health.

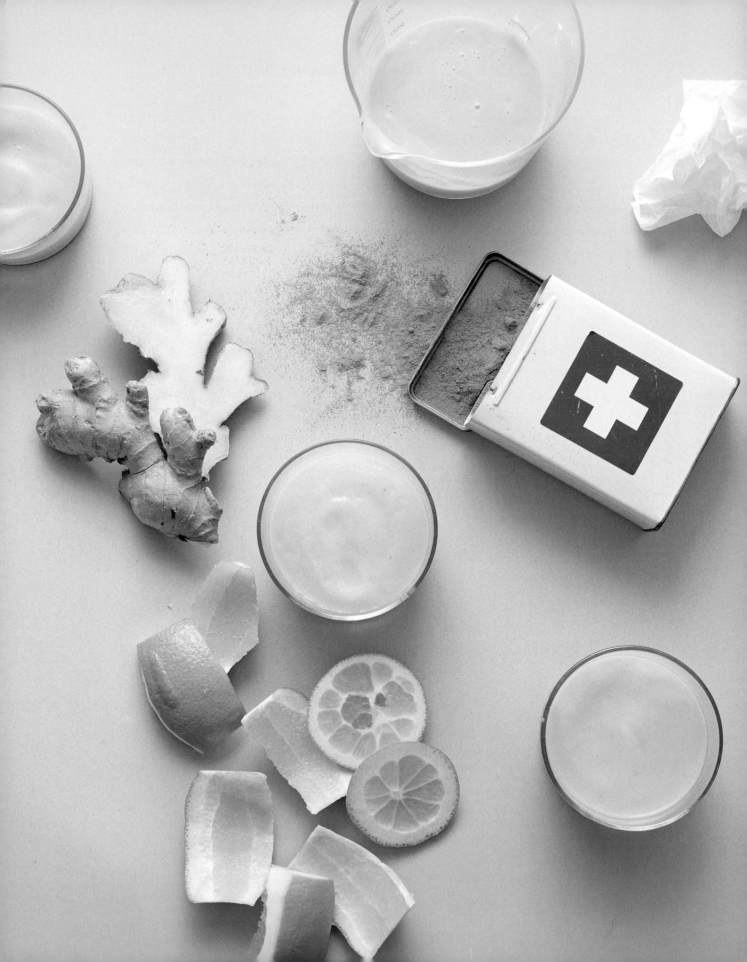

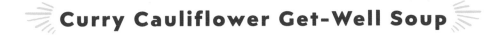

Curry Cauliflower Get-Well Soup

This was the final recipe I created for this book because one month before my deadline, I suffered from a brutal twenty-six-day cold. By far, the worst cold of my life. This cold was so bad that I fully lost my sense of smell and taste. I couldn't tell this curry soup from ketchup soup. Now that I can taste again, let me confirm that these flavors are otherworldly, as is the texture if you're into thick creamy soup. If you're not, don't puree everything with the immersion blender, so you have thin broth with heartier bits.

SERVES ABOUT 6

1 large head of cauliflower, washed and chopped

2 tablespoons olive oil

Sea salt or pink salt

¾ cup quinoa, any color

1 yellow onion, chopped

2 or 3 garlic cloves, chopped

1 medium sweet potato, chopped

2 or 3 tablespoons Thai red curry paste (read the ingredients to make sure the one you're buying doesn't contain fish sauce if you don't eat that)

½ teaspoon ground ginger or 1½ teaspoons peeled and chopped fresh

½ teaspoon ground turmeric

1½ cups veggie broth

1 14-ounce can lite coconut milk or 14 ounces almond milk

1 tablespoon freshly squeezed lime juice

Fresh cilantro, chopped, to taste, for garnish

Pumpkin seeds, for garnish

1. Preheat the oven to 400°F.
2. Place the cauliflower in a large bowl. Drizzle with 1 tablespoon of the olive oil and a hefty sprinkle of salt and toss around so the cauliflower is evenly coated.
3. Transfer the cauliflower to a rimmed baking sheet and roast in the oven for 30 minutes or until the tips of the cauliflower are golden brown.
4. While the cauliflower is roasting, cook the quinoa by rinsing it and adding it to a small saucepan with 1½ cups of water. Cover it, bring it to a boil, and then remove the lid and reduce the heat to a light simmer.
5. In a large pot over medium heat, add the remaining 1 tablespoon olive oil, the onion, garlic, and a generous pinch of salt. Sauté, stirring occasionally, for about 3 minutes, until the onion and garlic turn soft and translucent.

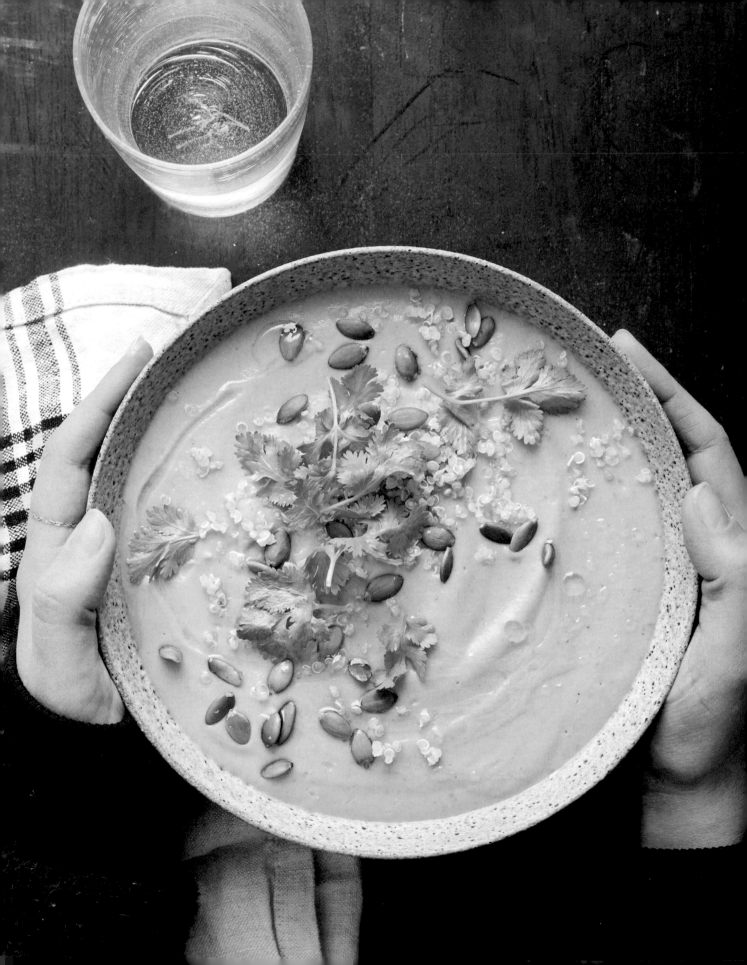

6. Add the sweet potato, curry paste, ginger, and turmeric, stir to incorporate, and cook for 3 more minutes.

7. Add the cauliflower, veggie broth, and coconut milk and bring to a light boil. Reduce the heat to low and let the mixture simmer for 10 minutes, until the sweet potato is soft when you stab it with a fork. Turn off the heat.

8. When the soup has cooled somewhat, add the lime juice and ½ teaspoon salt. Use an immersion blender to puree it right in the pot. If you don't have an immersion blender, use a ladle to transfer it to a high-speed blender (only filling the blender about halfway) and blend until creamy. Pour into a serving bowl and repeat until you've pureed all the soup.

9. Pour the soup into serving bowls and add ¼ to ½ cup of quinoa to each. Garnish with chopped cilantro.

AFTER [PARTY] THOUGHT:

Add even more veggies to this party pot at the end of cooking,
such as sautéed, steamed, or roasted chopped peppers, zucchini,
and spinach.

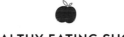

HEALTHY EATING ~~SUCKS~~:

"I feel like when most people think of the word 'soup,'
they don't think of it as a filling meal. At least I don't. This soup,
however, is so filling and delicious and so hearty!"
—BL

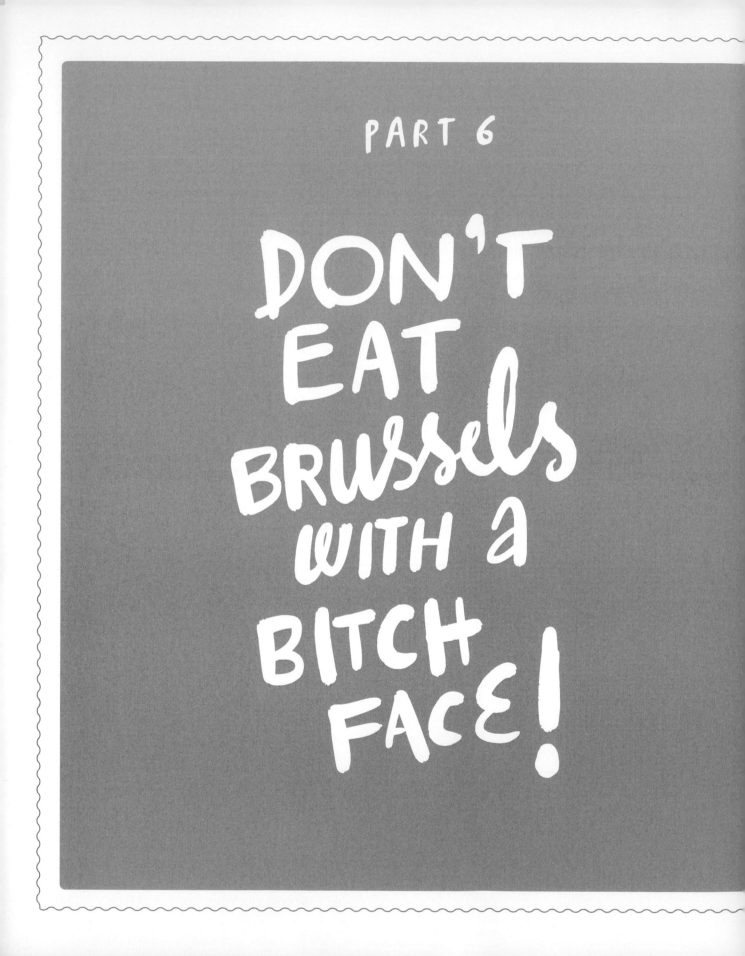

PART 6

DON'T EAT BRUSSELS WITH a BITCH FACE!

(please)

This is the part of the book where it's, well, over. This is the end. It's time to stop drooling over these recipes and go make them. For real, don't just stick a Post-it on the ones that look good and put the book on your shelf. I didn't write this thing to be a hammock for your dust! I'd rather you drip pesto on one page, spill some matcha latte on another, and light part three on fire sautéing spinach. Walk that cutie booty into the kitchen and *cook something, now.* (Said with love.)

And after that? Consciously continue sliding more crap off and edging more plants onto your plates. Or bowls. Or mugs, fistfuls, even cocktails.

Plant-partying is not a fad, my friend. Even though it might be trending on Instagram or magazine stands, it is *not* a fad. Because fads go out of fad, and eating a diet of primarily plants will never not be fab. You keep eating Brussels without a bitch face and the only thing that will become dull is not feeling, looking, and living your best.

It's all good. Relax, smile, play pickup Frisbee, binge *Game of Thrones,* throw your dog a bone, travel to Thailand, kiss that girl, try improv, run a glow-in-the-dark 5K, feng shui your nightstand; you'll have the energy to do it all if you eat more plants. With a smile.

Acknowledgments

It took many a "gracious loser's face" moments to get to this moment where I get to write my own book's acknowledgments page.

Kids, if you're watching at home, don't give up. Don't ever give up on your dream. Back in 2008, when I was sitting on the floor at that place that rhymes with "Darnes and Toble" taking manic handwritten notes from books sorta like this, optimistic but unsure about my potential for a better, healthier, happier life, I really didn't know it'd be *actually* possible to one day be the author of a book about such life that ideally, you actually purchased. I want to thank YOU a million kale bunches for doing that.

Additionally, I am up to my ears in gratitude for:

My PIMPbassadors, because of whom this process felt like a party. Without all 147 of you, creating this book would've been much more *The Shining*, instead of the *Bridesmaides* that it was. Also without you, the chai banana bread wouldn't be nearly chai-y enough and the caulifredo recipe would be a pain in the ass. Thank you for bringing my kitchen creations into your homes and into the mouths of your loved ones. To the superstars who tested a mega-amount of recipes: April Say, Alena Purvis, Alexa Karp, Allison Goldin, Amanda Hopper, Andrea Romesser, Anna Comes, Anna Dursztman, Becca Weidle, Blaise Lallathin, BreAnne Knapik, Brittany O'Connor, Caprice Sola, Cassie Bolden, Catherine Ashworth, Chelsea Donahue, Corri Carpenter, Franki Amro, Gabrielle Howard, Gianna Dinuzzo, Hannah Belle Solomon, Holly Greenberg, Isabella Dawes, Jane Murphy, Jenna Nelson, Jennifer Stefancik, Jenny Palacio, Jenny Walrod, Jessica Cobian, Jessica Jackson, Jessica Rothman, Juliana Hart, Kaitlin Parker, Kalin Haley, Karen Brady, Katie Thompson, Kierin Maloney, Kimberly Springer, Lauren Gordon, Lisa Brooks, Mandi Donaldson, Mattie Canaday, Megan Hillman, Melanie Muskus, Melissa Lalonde, Rebecca Adelson, Rhyan Geiger, Samantha Bush, Nicole Rosalyn Sheynin, Sara Drummond, Sarah Davis, Sasha Rashid, Taylor Zele, Valerie Kasper, Victoria Casenhiser, truly couldn't have done this without you. "Thank you" scratches the surface and "Let's do it again ASAP" tells the truth!

My photo team, who became my family, my appreciation and admiration of you is endless. Take every bark Tommy had over our unforgettable two weeks and replace each one with a "thank you" and you'd be close to where I'm at. My girl-band: Kate Buckens on the food styling; Maeve Sheridan on the props; and Linda Xiao on the camera, you are magic. Without you, this book would just be a photo of my hand. Drew, our unsung hero, my mind's still blown that you didn't even break a dish. And yes, everyone, I'm still eating leftovers.

Erin Fiore, that damn plant confetti was the best thing to ever happy to me! Thank you for illustrating all of the important things in my life, from my websites to my wedding invites to everything in this book; I'm endlessly grateful for how your pen puts my parties on paper.

Lindsay Edgecombe, I have eternal appreciation for you hoisting my literary dreams into reality. Thank you for being even-keeled when I was whatever the opposite sailing term for *even keel* is! Your endless encouragement, creativity, commitment, and belief in me has rocked my world and changed my life.

Nina Shield, I'll never forget the evening after our first phone call, swooning to Jesse over a big bowl'o pasta with plants about how badly I wanted to work with you. I'm so blessed the feeling was mutual. (It's okay if the swooning part was not.) Thank you for letting this book stay real; editing it but not altering me, igniting my love affair with the thesaurus, and for letting me keep 40 of the 800+ exclamation points I tried to sneak into this book!!! (Now 43. Ha.) You are the best and you made my first book-birthing process the best—wait! thesaurus: You made my first book-birthing process outstanding, first-rate, aces.

Lorie Pagnozzi, you rock! So much thanks for your so much excitement for this book! I'm tremendously fortunate to have had your enthusiasm and commitment to conveying my energy via design.

Shelby Meizlik, I'll never forget your initial belief in me. You gave me the courage to open my wings and fly, even if I ended up flying out of a different coordinate. Thank you, thank you.

Terry Walters, thanks for paving the plant-eating path from my backyard and pushing me to "Absolutely get an agent, are you crazy?!" and for your tempeh recipe on page 165.

Shannon Kaiser, thank you for teaching me that rejection is protection and that following joy can never leave you lost.

Christine Clifton, thank you for you helping me continually throw my BS in my food disposal.

Sloane, everyone needs that friend who "thinks Skittles count as fruit" and I'm so lucky you're mine. Thanks for your dietarily unconditional friendship. Your hand looks great grabbing that date on page 142.

In loving memory of Nancy, who preferred pork to plants but would've championed this book as much as anyone. I miss sharing meals with you.

Nina, who really had nothing to do with this book but has everything to do with being the best sister on the planet. Actually, scratch that, you do have a lot to do with this book since I essentially wrote it for you. Maybe someday you'll look back and realize your big sis was right (as per usual) and start pumping your body with plants. Until then, I'll always cook for you. Love you more than words.

Mom and Dad, who embraced my radical diet change like it was your own. At least around me. There's a zero percent chance PIMP would exist without you. Thanks for helping me through my rock bottoms and hugging me at the mountaintops. Thank you for cheerleading my comedy sets, my crying seasons, and my clean eating. Thank you for giving my business cards to people you eavesdrop on in restaurants and on golf courses. "I love you" doesn't even cut it close.

Jesse, you were my missing ingredient. Without you, I'd only have plants. Thank you for putting the party in my life and helping me stay well enough to keep that party going. Thank you for believing in me, never letting me quit, and constantly cleaning out our fridge, which is what you're doing right now as I type this. I'm honored to get to party with you for the rest of our lives, which hopefully is a very long time thanks to all the kale we eat. (Yes, I recycled that part from my wedding vows.) I love you to all the moons.

Index

Note: Page numbers in *italics* indicate recipe photos separate from recipe text.

ingredients. *See also specific main ingredients*
    basic. *See* basic bitches: freezer items, 31–32
    for fridge, 35
    for pantry/dry goods storage, 33–34, 36
    reading between food label lines, 37–38
    real estate lesson, 39
    trendy foods and, 30
    "would-be-nice-ables," 35–36

J

jars, glass, 42
Jesse's Secret Creamy, Dreamy Pumpkin
    Oatmeal, 84–85

K

kale
    All the Fall Feels Salad, 161–62
    Dr. Oz Said . . . This Kale Mint Chocolate Chip
        Ice Cream, So . . . , 156–*59*
    Nacho-Unhealthy Nachos, *192*–93
    other recipes with, 59–63, *104*–6, *184*–85
    Staples R US Tahini TeriyakYAY Bowl, 119–*20*
    There's an "I" in Buffalo Cauliflower Dip,
        241–42
    The "Too Good to Have a Fear of Heights"
        Green Sandie, 252–*53*
kettle corn, cinnamon, 226
kitchen tools, 41–42
kombucha
    about: appeal/benefits of, 246–47
    about, detoxing with cocktails of, 246–47
    'Bucha Mule, 155
    Fauxmosas, 186

L

labels, reading between the lines, 37–38
leafy greens, to stock, 31
leftovers, making them bestovers, 100–102
lemon and lime. *See* citrus
listening to your body, 11, 309–10

M

mango, snacks with, *172*–73, *224*–25
Maple Mustard Dressing, 161
matcha
    about
        Banana Ice Cream with, 110
        Chia Pudding with, 28
        Overnight Oats with, 116
    Banana Ice Cream with, 110–*11*
    Matcha Mint Chocolate Chip Energy Balls,
        275
    Mix-and-Match-a Matcha Latte, 276–77

milk, nondairy
    about
        easy dairy swaps, 51
        lattes with, 3, 229–30, 276–77
        to stock, 31
    Hot Golden Milk, 228
mint
    about: Banana Ice Cream with chocolate chip
        and, 110
    Dr. Oz Said . . . This Kale Mint Chocolate Chip
        Ice Cream, So . . . , 156–*59*
    Matcha Mint Chocolate Chip Energy Balls,
        275
miso
    about: nutritional benefits and uses, 35
    Tahini Miso Magic Sauce, 273
movies, snacks for, 223–26
    about: overview of, 223
    Decked-Out Cinnamon Kettle Corn, 226
    Super-Fun Mango Sriracha Popcorn Mix,
        224–*25*
Muhammara May I, 232–*33*
mulled wine, 168
mushrooms
    about: healing ability of, 326
    Beats Meat Balls (Mushroom-Lentil Balls),
        62–63
    Weeknight-Friendly Fajitas, 68–*71*

N

nachos, 87, *192*–93
nutrient density, 204
nutritional yeast, 36, 44
nuts and seeds
    about
        eating more plants, 286, 287
        protein in, 44
        to stock, 34
        volume control, 286
    All the Fall Feels Salad, 161–62
    Banana Cream Pie, 150–51
    Banana Ice Cream with, 110–12
    Better Than a Snickers Bar Bites, 141–*42*
    Cashew Sour Cream, 68–69
    Cashew Sweet Cream, 203–4
    Chia Pudding, *288*–89
    Curry Car Cashews, 257
    Gift-Worthy Granola, *262*–64
    Heaven in My Apartment Protein Smoothie,
        296–97
    Lemon Chia–Not–Poppy Seed Mini Muffins,
        81–*83*
    Liquid Gold Cheese Sauce, 55
    Muhammara May I, 232–*33*
    My Besto Planty Pesto Formula, 212
    Nice Crispy Treats, 197–98